THE NATURE OF CLINICAL CARE

VOLUME 2

Mental Health and Public Health Care

by

David Zitner and H. Dominic J. Covvey

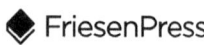

FriesenPress

One Printers Way
Altona, MB R0G 0B0
Canada

www.friesenpress.com

ISBN
978-1-03-918858-7 (Hardcover)
978-1-03-918857-0 (Paperback)
978-1-03-918859-4 (eBook)

1. MEDICAL, HEALTH CARE DELIVERY

Distributed to the trade by The Ingram Book Company

Dedications and Credits

DAVID:

My family, patients and students taught me most of what I know. Friends and family motivated me and organized my thinking. Neil Roberts, CEO of the Halifax Infirmary, John Ruedy, Dean of Medicine at Dalhousie, and Brian Lee Crowley, CEO MacDonald Laurier Institute diverted me from clinical practice to research and teaching. My students showed me that people who understand the basic ideas in Medicine as discussed in these books could solve many simple and complex medical problems and more easily collaborate with clinicians.

DOMINIC:

Over 7 years ago, David invited me to co-write a book with him. His success in his Health Informatics course at Dalhousie University motivated his belief that similar material could benefit others. I accepted and enjoyed hundreds of highly stimulating phone discussions that underpin this Compendium. Thank you David! Thanks also to Elisabeth and Henry! I am the lucky dog who got the excellent attention they provide to pets and other animals. Finally, to Natela, Zaza, Lizi and Tina, whom Putin displaced. Слава Україні! Героям слава! You too are heroes!

CREDITS:

Dominic's daughter, Laura S. Thompson, painted the cover image. She and her husband, Frank Rekrut, are artists with an art school in Florence, Italy (www.theflorencestudio.com). Dominic's younger daughter, Beth A. Covvey, illustrated this and the other Volumes. Learn about her work at www.bethcovvey.ca. Beth lives in Yellowknife, Northwest Territory, Canada. Thanks also to Brittany Kraus for addressing the many issues in the books! Brittany, you were a lucky find!

Comment

Our goal in producing these books was affordability. Several publishers quoted well over $100 USD for each volume. So, we opted for less expensive electronic publishing and minimal royalties. We would welcome any error-finds and suggestions regarding content so we can improve the text. You can share with us via we.inform.people@gmail.com.

Table of Contents

VOLUME 2

—————————— Section 1 ——————————

INTRODUCTION

DOCTOR VS DOCTOR

In every profession there are friendly rivalries among specialists. It's the same in health care.

A GP, internist, surgeon, and a pathologist are out one day duck hunting. First up is the GP who takes aim at a flock of birds passing overhead and says, "Looks like a duck, flies like a duck, quacks like a duck, it must be a duck." BANG! And the GP bags a duck.

The internist then steps up, takes aim at a 2nd flock of birds flying overhead. Says, "Looks like a duck, flies like a duck, quacks like a duck, rule out quail, rule out pheasant, goose versus duck likely." BANG! And bags a duck.

A 3rd flock of birds then flies overhead and the surgeon steps up and starts shooting at the flock. BANG! BANG! BANG! BANG! And dead birds are dropping all around. The surgeon lowers the gun, walks over to one of the dead birds, picks one up, hands it to the pathologist and says, "Tell me if this is a duck."

Based on Wolfescape Medical Humor - http://www.wolfescape.com/Humour/MedJokes.htm#Top

A Story:

A 30-year-old athletic woman was outraged when she realized that her doctor had effectively lied to her. She had gone to the doctor because she felt tired, worn down and unmotivated. At her visit, she was told that she had a disease, which the doctor said was "Depression" caused by a "biochemical abnormality". The doctor had ordered some tests and prescribed an antidepressant, which she filled at the pharmacy and took for the first month before seeing her doctor again. When she went for her next visit, she learned her laboratory test results came back as totally normal. Being an intelligent patient, she decided to gradually wean herself off the antidepressant medication, took up an exercise program, was careful with her diet, and hoped her fatigue would end. Sure enough, soon she felt fine without the medication and this caused her to realize that her fatigue was just a consequence of her busy lifestyle that had distracted her from caring for herself and getting adequate sleep.

Chapter 1: —————— A Preface

Many books describe the health system. This compendium of books, though, is unique. We commence our story in Volume 1 with the nature of the clinical process – what doctors do – and reflect on the clinical process as the source of information that serves as the foundation from which every aspect of health care devolves, from caring for patients to evaluating the value of medical investigations, treatments and the care agencies themselves. We examine many aspects and styles of practice, especially from the perspective of patients. In this volume we go beyond physical health and deal with mental health and Public Health. A consistent theme throughout the material is patient engagement in care so the patient is understood to be a crucial operational agent in the system. These books provide the perspectives of clinicians, informaticians and patients, being strongly shaped by the background of its authors.

What You Have in Hand ——————

Everyone participating in health care must comprehend a set of essential ideas.

There are three books in this series. Volume 1 introduces the ideas related to understanding, diagnosing, treating, and preventing biological problems. Volume 2 applies those ideas, enabling the reader to understand Public Health and Mental Health. Volume 3 reflects on important issues that underly the practice of clinical care.

You can read the chapters in each book in order, or it is possible to skip around and read the material relevant to your needs at the time and to your background. However, each chapter is a kind of 'microbook' that can be read on its own. We have attempted to write the chapters so there is little essential dependence on other material. Where we believe that understanding something is enhanced by or dependent on by other material, we have stated such. Though scientific articles are usually written in a highly structured way and build up a story, many scientists read their contents in different orders. Richard Feynman, the famous Nobel Laureate, was known to often read only the introductory abstract of an article, then read the conclusions, then work it all out in his head and only go through the rest if he came to different conclusions. So, you see, to each, your own!

There are 3 books with over 85 chapters divided up into the 3 volumes. We will include this same **Introduction** in each of the volumes, thereby assisting in our 'start anywhere- go anywhere' approach!

Note that this material is available online or printed.

Why Consider these Books ——————

We assume you thought that one or more of these books looked interesting because you picked them from a list, the Web or a shelf and began reading them. Nevertheless, might they really be of value to you or your students?

There are many texts on Medicine or that address various aspects of health care, but this compendium is different. It unseals and unwraps what we call the 'health care system' (though many would deny that it is organized well enough that we should call it a 'system') enabling a deep understanding of its nature, parts, people and functions. In a way, these books describe the anatomy (parts and connections) and physiology (functions) of the health system. They describe the professionals that make the system work and what they do, as well as the strengths, weaknesses and flaws of every important aspect – their pathology. Most importantly, the ideas support collaborations of health professionals with each other and between patients and health care teams.

This compendium of books describes the most important concepts that medical professionals – clinicians (physicians, nurses and allied care providers) – use to assess, diagnose and treat problems. It explains how clinicians think, the kinds of information they use to reach conclusions, how they decide to treat and what they can and cannot do. Those ideas will give readers, including teachers and students in many disciplines, the understanding, skills and confidence to themselves find pertinent health information and will enable nonclinical healthcare professionals and patients to understand the clinical process and to have intelligent conversations with clinicians about their work.

The material might surprise the reader by revealing that not all recommended medical tests or treatments are necessarily good ones that they should accept. It will, on the other hand, also suggest how to decide when it is appropriate to accept or reject suggestions that a problem is not real or is "unimportant" and therefore not requiring tests or treatments. Readers will realize that medical care is powerful but has limits. We try to identify beliefs that lead people to accept useless and possibly harmful care or to agree with incomplete or mistaken diagnoses or inappropriate treatments.

After reading the books in this series, the reader will know the most important ideas that clinicians use. That will give the confidence and skills to find and understand pertinent health information, converse with and about clinicians, and understand how patients can become active participants in their own and their families' health care.

Beyond all that, these books will help the reader understand what it means to be healthy and how patients can help physicians[1] keep them as healthy as possible. In addition, they will help readers understand the origins of controversies in health services administration and prepare them to contribute to the discussion.

Why Develop Health Literacy and Engage Patients

On September 22nd, 2011, the now-defunct Health Council of Canada released *"How Engaged are Canadians in their Primary Care? Results from the 2010 Commonwealth Fund International Health Policy Survey"* and reported that fewer than half (48%) of all Canadians are active participants in their own health care.[2] We are fairly sure that this is the case in most other jurisdictions.

The Commonwealth Fund study found that engaged patients are happier with their care and more likely to participate in disease prevention, in appropriate screening and in health promoting activities. It has become clear that modern technology enables everyone, clinicians and non-clinicians alike, to work together to achieve better health and better treatment.

---

[1] Note: We will refer to the role 'physician' throughout these books to avoid cumbersome language and because physicians have a broader scope of practice, including an almost unlimited ability to order tests and treatments. Other clinicians (nurses and allied professionals) might carry out similar functions, but their scope of practice is more limited. We recognize that all members of the healthcare team are vital, and that many clinicians who are not physicians have unique and essential roles and expertise.

[2] How Engaged are Patients in Their Primary Care. https://secure.cihi.ca/free_products/CMWF_Bulletin_5_EN.pdf. Accessed December 7, 2022.

The World Health Organization[3] reports that several interventions help non-clinicians (including patients, administrators and regulators) become more health literate and able to play an active role in their own care. This is important, as **health-literate patients feel comfortable in shared decision-making** because they feel confident in evaluating professional suggestions. Health-literate patients are better able to recognize when self-management is appropriate and when they need advice. FIGURE 2.1.1 illustrates that patients and physicians must work together.

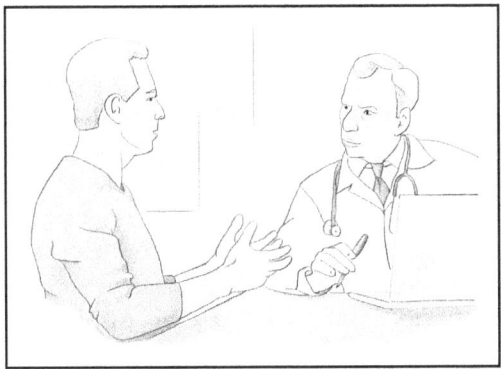

FIGURE 2.1.1: Patient and Clinician Working Together

Health literacy improves when patients have access to:

> Written information that supplements clinical consultations.

> Web sites and other electronic information sources.

> Personalized computer-based information and virtual support.

> Decision aids for patients.

> Self-management education programs including the ideas in these volumes.

The fact is that ordinary people can easily find information on the causes of many health problems and on the effectiveness of treatments if they know where to look and what questions to ask.

Why Health Professionals Need Similar Information

Health services administrators, health informaticians and other health care-interested professionals need the same information as patients and their care providers. Administrators, for instance, need information about the effectiveness of care to evaluate the services that they manage and support. Journalists need that information so they can inform the public. In addition, Health Informatics (See Volume 1 Chapter 19) experts must know about the kinds of information that clinicians produce or collect during care and how they and researchers use or should use it. Clinical information is the essential content of health information systems intended to assess care and inform clinicians and administrators about the benefits and harms of care.

Artificial Intelligence

IBM's Big Blue long ago beat two contestants in *Jeopardy*. Then another computer, using artificial intelligence (AI[4], also called 'Machine Intelligence') defeated an expert in the complicated game *Go*, a game requiring knowledge and strategy. There is the promise that those same artificial intelligence techniques can help clinicians and patients make better choices as they try to diagnose what is wrong with the patient and attempt to decide the best way to treat both common and rare health problems.

Artificial intelligence systems process vast amounts of information and discover the relationships among various pieces of information. People who develop and use artificial

---

3   https://www.researchgate.net/publication/238728706_Where_are_the_Patients_in_Decision-Making_About_Their_Own_Care; https://www.who.int/publications/i/item/9789240039872. Accessed December 7, 2022.

4   https://www.theguardian.com/technology/2016/jan/27/google-hits-ai-milestone-as-computer-beats-go-grandmaster. Accessed December 7, 2022.

intelligence systems to support health care must understand the knowledge base and principles of health care to select meaningful information and to evaluate if the conclusions produced by AI systems are meaningful and correct.

In Volume 1 Chapter 4, we discuss distinctions between the art of Medicine and the science of Medicine. Artificial intelligence methods rely on machines having access to massive amounts of scientific information to discover relationships among patient characteristics, healthcare activities and results. However, at this stage of development, artificial intelligence systems are less useful when it comes to the art of Medicine. They are impaired in inferring suggestions when the information and research is insufficient to reach a scientific conclusion, although AI system may help scientists help develop testable ideas (hypotheses) that can be supported or rejected by additional research.

Whenever clinicians differ on the approach to problems, patients and clinicians must have the knowledge and tools to help decide among different possibilities, especially when the science backing choices is limited.

The Importance of Health ───────

We all worry, from time to time, about our health, even when we are well. We may worry even more when we do not feel right, when something hurts, or when we are unable to do what we were able to do before.

There is no question that most important regarding our health is how we feel about ourselves – that we are reasonably content with ourselves – our nature. This even applies to those of us who might have experienced the exigencies of aging (cataracts, for instance), or lost a limb, endured paralysis or function despite some other challenge.

However, the next concern is for how well we and those close to us feel, think, function, and, sometimes, how long we and they are likely to be around. Health is right up there near the top of each of our lists. Like it or not, our health affects every day of our lives and every hour of each of those days. Further, what we do on those days affects our health.

Some of us get through life with few health problems. But that's not true of all of us and we each know of someone not so lucky. A certainty is that all of us will from time to time get sick, sometimes very sick and eventually mortally sick. In other words, we will die.

Regarding our health, there are many questions.

What exactly do we mean by 'being healthy' and what do we mean by 'being sick'? What do we need to do to keep us healthy and what do clinicians need to do to help us when we're sick? How can we contribute and help clinical teams help us? Who are those people who do the helping? What are their and our responsibilities related to health both for ourselves and for others? What is the system that tries to help us remain healthy and that treats us when are sick, and how does it work? What is a 'diagnosis' and what information is necessary to make a diagnosis? What are the kinds of things we can do to maintain health, avoid and treat illness? Why do some treatments, intended to help us, fail or hurt us? Why do other treatments sometimes magically work? Why is everything the way it is, the human body, the care providers, the healthcare system, the treatments, and the effects they deliver? What information is needed to predict whether a treatment is more likely to help or to harm? Why is mental illness controversial? What are the differences between problems that we call 'illnesses' and those we label 'mental illness'?

We answer all these questions and many more in these volumes.

Most people will find the ideas we present compelling and easy to understand. People who understand the important ideas can better understand most clinical information, accept useful suggestions, and discard harmful ones. People who know the important ideas will also find it easier to access the information they need to guide their professional, personal and political choices for health care.

Eventually, all of us make healthcare choices. Clinicians ask us to opine on healthcare interventions for ourselves, for friends and for family. At the ballot box, politicians ask us to choose the best proposals for organizing health care. Health is an important part of life and touches everyone and everything.

So, we have a lot to learn. What's important is that health knowledge will empower us!

Chapter 2: ——— Welcome to Our Readers

This is a condensed version of several introductory chapters in Volume 1. We intend it to provide a framework for reading the material that follows.

The material in this compendium is meant for many different groups of readers, including those participating in, studying, evaluating, reporting on, administering, or in any other way becoming involved with the healthcare system. However, everyone can understand them. The important ideas herein include:

> The purposes of health care.

> How we can measure and assess the impact of health care.

> What Preventive Medicine and screening for undiagnosed problems are about.

> What diagnosis involves and how it determines the presence of absence of disease.

> How doctors interpret and use the results of diagnostic tests and procedures.

> Why some medical test results for a disease produce false alarms or misleading reassurance.

> What the value, benefits and harms are of certain treatments.

> How we can use tests and treatments to avoid illness and maintain health.

> What the purposes and problems of treatments in mental health are.

> What the major healthcare controversies in diagnosis, treatment and screening are.

These volumes are primarily for non-clinical professionals who work in or interact with the healthcare system. These include patients, as well as health informaticians and health information managers (medical records librarians), technicians and technologists, health services administrators, journalists, pharmaceutical company representatives, politicians, lawyers, judges and insurance company leadership and staff. Informaticians work with medical information. Lawyers interact with patients and the healthcare system – assessing claims of medical damage or injury and the interpreting what the causes and effects of injuries are. Judges address health care-related lawsuits, and drug and insurance company personnel sell or apply their products and services within the healthcare enterprise. Technicians and technologists use equipment in care processes. Last, but not least, we have kept in mind journalists and other writers, who must understand the nature and practice (and vocabulary) of medical care and be able to interpret and report on medical research results and claims about interventions.

To collaborate with non-clinicians as well as other medical professionals, clinicians must share compatible understandings of the purposes of care, hold harmonious ideas around general and specific approaches to clinical problems and agree on how to resolve differences of opinion among team members. They will also benefit from this material.

The Function of this Compendium

The reader will find that this compendium is like medical care itself. Much of what we discuss is based on scientific evidence, while other things represent what people call the 'art of Medicine', a necessary and valuable part of clinical care. The reader will learn how to tell the difference between conclusions based on medical science and those which, necessarily, are based on the art of Medicine.

We will show how the parts of the health-care system work – and sometimes do not – and what their good and bad effects are. We also will discuss the magic of medical care. That magic sometimes hides behind the 'placebo effect'. Some even call these magical effects 'miracles'. So, we will approach the material a bit scientifically and a bit artistically. This is appropriate, as both the science and the art are crucial, and it is important to understand when conclusions are based on art, and when on science.

The Expectations on the Reader

Because we intended these books for many audiences, we have tried to define every term and present material clearly and succinctly. It is our bad if any ideas seem obscure. Nothing is truly complicated in these books. The important ideas are easy to understand and do not require sophisticated backgrounds. However, there are a few more-challenging sections. Even there, readers can understand the important ideas without deep knowledge of the underlying concepts, but those who want to go deeper can access the references. The truth is that we have not expected readers to be anything more than curious.

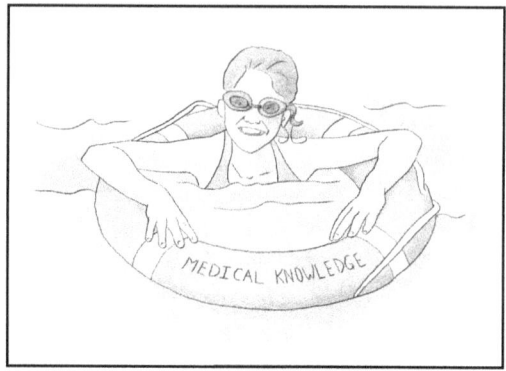

FIGURE 2.2.1: Medical Knowledge Can Be a Life Preserver

Medical Knowledge as Life Saving (See FIGURE 2.2.1)

Another reason these books are important is the ideas in them can save lives. The content enables patients to avoid preventable medical errors.

Some interventions undertaken in health care can have disastrous impacts. Medicines can kill. Even skilled surgeons leave some patients either permanently injured or dead. Screening tests, meant to prevent illness, sometimes initiate a cascade of ill-advised follow-up procedures and treatments. The result can be that people trying to prevent illness, experience injury rather than benefit.

We show how to make decisions about submitting to testing or undertaking a treatment. We try to inform good decisions based on real facts about the chances that testing or treatment will help or harm.

The knowledge herein encourages sensible and appropriate participation in the care process. The buzz-phrase today is 'patient engagement', meaning that patients work **with** their care providers to make good choices. Remember that the patient is the one gambling that an intervention will help, not harm.

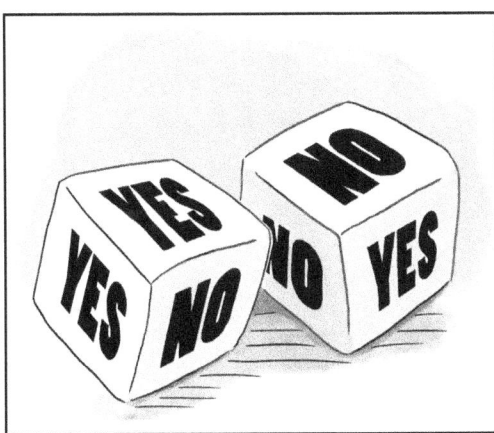

FIGURE 2.2.2: Rolling the Dice – Taking a Chance

In movies a surgeon might say: "I'm going to take the risk…". However, it's the patient who takes the risk! See FIGURE 2.2.2. So, the patient must decide whether or not to accept a physician's recommendation. We discuss the real meaning of 'informed consent' to treatment. Perhaps it would be clearer if we said that patients are the Chief Executive Officers of their bodies and the physician is a consultant! The final responsibility is and must be with the patient. It used to be that many saw the doctor as a kind of demigod, and the patient was supposed to be an obedient disciple. But that's no longer the case, because no one endows medical school graduates with omnipotent competencies and we all can access medical information.

The authors have spent their lives trying to help people realize that health care is a 'team sport', an interactive relationship between knowledgeable care providers and informed patients, the central team of health care. On any team, all must have the competence to be independent, but work together.

We provide the knowledge everybody needs to participate in health care. Without that knowledge we are clued-out amateurs trying to play football not knowing the rules, how football works, what to do, and what the goals of the game are. Our objective is to turn "players" in the healthcare "game" into competent players. You will see that health care is an exciting process where people often make important wagers whose outcome is crucial to their health and well-being.

Promoting Empowerment is a Major Goal

We believe that readers and those they affect can, armed with these ideas, understand empowerment and become empowered. These books, though, focus their efforts on making readers deeply aware of the nature of health, health care and the health system, as this provides the foundation for empowerment. We think immersing oneself in the content of the books being like entering basic training in the military. The recruit learns about the instruments of warfare, the importance of fitness and how to get there and stay there. In boot camp the military transforms ordinary people into fighting units, where working as a cohesive team to overcome an enemy becomes even more important than staying alive. The knowledge in these books can effect transitions like this in the reader, albeit for peaceful and defensive purposes. In health care, becoming part of a cohesive team can help people feel better, improve their function and stay alive.

These books will also give a new perception of the healthcare system, of care providers and of what patient-physician collaboration requires. They will help the reader to make good decisions or to coach others how to do that. These decisions are the 'weapons' for dealing with health care and its professionals. We will tell the truth and some of the truths will likely be surprising – and some may be a bit difficult to swallow. However, it is the truth and with that truth, people can improve and protect their lives.

The Results We Expect

So, we have written what this set of books is all about, what the content can do, why people need to absorb it and what they can do with it.

We are convinced that the knowledge learned will reduce medical errors, save people from injury and death, reduce the cost of the healthcare system, and potentiate a longer, more comfortable life. And, importantly, one with less worry.

Chapter 3: ——— Our Promises and Overview

Promises, promises! Here they are.

Promise 1: We shall dissect the anatomy and describe the function of healthcare system, define human health and sickness and reveal the nature of medical care (both the art and science thereof).

Promise 2: We will define every term and explain things as clearly as possible clearly.

Promise 3: We will offer knowledge that can save lives.

Promise 4: Our most important promise is to provide sufficient information to facilitate participation in care.

Promise 5: In a way, we have promised to surprise.

Promise 6: We will try to keep your attention, sometimes with anecdotes from our or others' experience.

Hopefully readers will agree that we have delivered on these promises after we finally drag them into the books.

Some of the Key Ideas in this Compendium ———

If readers ever find themselves taking on a challenge similar to writing books like these, they will probably get sucked into thinking, as we have, that every word is important. Unfortunately, for a few readers some words may prove to be too many, too few or the wrong ones. Today, be by news organizations, many

have come to expect tiny parcels of knowledge and minimalist texts. Some won't want to read all the way through the books; others will wish for some kind of Reader's Digest-like summary.

However, we hope that our division of the material into many (almost a hundred) topical chapters should appeal to those seeking a more enjoyable 'tapas' approach to learning.

We hope you have read or will read Volume 1 on Physical Medicine, as it contains the foundation for the material in this volume. Even if you scan that volume, that will help. There is nothing in this one that is not understandable on its own, but topics like what health and disease are all about, the nature of the medical visit, the examination of the patient, diagnosis, treatment and follow-up will serve as a backdrop for understanding similar matters related to mental health care.

Bon Appétit!

VOLUME 2

Section 2

MENTAL HEALTH

IN PSYCHIATRY, HUMOR CAN REALLY HELP

Q: How many psychiatrists does it take to change a light bulb?
A: Just one, but the light bulb has to really want to change

Mr. Jones is in bad shape, so he goes to a psychiatrist. He tells his doctor: "I am suicidal and I need help! What shall I do?" His doctor responds: "I can try to help but you have to pay me in advance!"

A Very Old One (origin unknown):

Psychiatrist to patient: "What seems to be your problem?"

Patient to psychiatrist: "Well for a long time now I've believed that I'm really a dog!"
Psychiatrist to patient: "How long have you felt that way?"
Patient to psychiatrist: "Ever since I was a puppy."

Another Oldie:

A patient visited a psychiatrist because he was obsessed with pornography. The doctor decided to do a test that would help the patient free-associate and maybe discover the causal factor. So, the psychiatrist told the patient to look at a few pictures. First the doctor showed the patient a drawing of a triangle and asked what the patient saw. The patient said: "That's a naked woman." "Wow!" the psychiatrist thought. The next drawing was of a square. The patient's response was the same: "A naked woman." "Holy mackerel!" thought the psychiatrist. The final drawing was of a circle and the patient again responded: "A naked woman." Floored by this response, the doctor said: "You really have a major psychiatric problem!" to which the patient replied: "What do you expect when you keep showing me dirty pictures!"

Stories of Mental Health Patients

Michael was surprised to learn that mental health care's actual goal is to influence how people think, feel and behave. He was also surprised to learn that, despite hundreds of labels in the psychiatry catalogue of problems (DSM-5), our understanding of mental health problems falls into only one of 3 categories. Problems could relate to (1) common and rare diagnosable medical illnesses, such as thyroid disease, which cause mental symptoms, (2) what we experience in our life contexts, or (3) unfortunately, our ignorance: the origin of many mental problems is just not known. He was astounded to realize that mental health diagnoses are merely descriptive, restating a person's symptoms as if they were diseases without revealing their cause. This changed his life, as Michael had been seeing a Psychiatrist, now had one of those DSM labels and had received a prescription to 'treat' it. After a lot of thought, he decided to find a therapist with whom he could explore the issues that were besetting his life. He did not fill the prescription.

Fred, on the other hand, was surprised to learn that after years of treatment with antidepressants for "Depression" his doctor discovered that Fred had Addison's disease, a treatable medical condition. His years of purchasing and taking inappropriate drugs and enduring their side effects were wasted. The doctor thought he knew that the sickness he termed 'Depression' was causing Fred's depressed feelings and had not searched more deeply for a treatable biological cause of Fred's problem.

Some mental health problems are somewhat innocuous… if irritating. Consider Mary, who had a long history of mental health problems. She, one day, came to the realization that she could always get a day off work if she complained that visual hallucinations had returned. Whenever she wanted a day off, she said "I am seeing things; there are angels all around!" Her boss always gave her the day, and despite her problems, she never harmed anyone and her work performance was otherwise terrific. Notwithstanding those days off, she remains more productive than many of her colleagues.

Mary's friend, Luther, was prescribed an antidepressant drug because he felt "bad". Subsequently, he complained of changes in sex drive, increased appetite and weight gain. He developed a tremor and his doctor gave him another drug to deal with 'tardive dyskinesia', a side effect of some psycho-active drugs. Luther stopped complaining about feeling bad because he now had a reason: weight gain, decreased libido and tremor. His activity decreased and his doctor told him that she had done what was acceptable in the circumstance. Luther now began to doubt he had chosen the right doctor!

Even tricky situations can work. Lola, an intelligent, fit, 34-year-old university math professor was attracted to her family doctor. She'd been his patient for 4 years, visiting him twice a year for routine health issues. One Friday morning she got up the courage to call his office and insisted on speaking to him directly. Unfortunately, he was with a patient, but he called her back later. Fortified with a bit of chutzpa, she invited him to dinner at her house. Somewhat as she expected, he rejected the offer, while trying to be nice about it. At her next visit, she asked him out again and he refused again, saying that although he liked her, it would be ethically inappropriate for him to date a patient. This steamed her! While she cooked dinner, she raged against the arrogance of a profession that thought relationships with customers or patients were somehow different or wrong! Not given to defeat, she waited a few days and called him again. When she spoke with him, she reminded him of her international reputation and her status as a full professor at the school. Cupid eventually managed to fire an effective arrow that pierced his protective shields, and he agreed to meet her at the local pub for a light dinner. That evening they had a wonderful time, decided to do it again, became and remained lovers, lived together, didn't marry and had 2 children. The nature of human relationships can be more powerful than the ethical bonds humans place on them!

Chapter 4: ———— Am I Crazy?

KEYWORDS: Psychiatry, Mental Health, Mental Illness, Interventions to Change Thoughts, Feelings and Behavior, Mind Versus Brain, Remedies for Mental Health Problems

ABSTRACT: Some mental health problems are associated with diagnosed biological diseases. For example, thyroid and adrenal problems have biological effects – that have detectable biomarkers – as well as mental health difficulties such as fatigue. Other mental health problems are not associated with biological problems. Though many speculate about the biological causes of mental health disturbances, in the absence of objective markers of disease, it is merely speculation. How clinicians understand mental health influences the treatment they are most likely to use. Absent a known medical disease, it is more appropriate to intervene using non-pharmacological methods. If these fail, then drugs may be appropriate. They should not be the first resort.

Our Experience of Mental Health

The anthropologist, Franz Boas, suggested that Eskimos (properly: Inuit) have more than 50 words for 'snow' and are better able to perceive differences between types of snow.[5] However, the difference between the number of words we have in English for snow or ice and those used by the Inuit relates to differences in language structure and not differences in perception.[6] [7] Inuit words have suffixes indicating various kinds of snow, like sleeting snow or crystalline snow. In English we use compound words to express those same entities. The discussion is important because it supports our belief that the words we use reflect our perceptions and also influence how we perceive the world. Perhaps, though, the focus on snow is more intense for the Inuit because there is so much ice in so many forms that many different words are useful for carefully describing reality.

Compare this to the fact that in English, we have on the order of 50 to 100 expressions to say that we believe that someone is not mentally 'right' or is crazy. To illustrate this, we have put a few of those below. Perhaps you can add to them from your experience.

IS IT BECAUSE WE SEE A LOT?

A polymath friend of DC's noticed we have many expressions for people whom we perceive as different mentally. The number of these words is large and only a few examples are below, as we listed close to 100:

– Insane
– One brick shy of a load
– Went nuts
– Strange
– Crazy
– Half bubble off plumb
– Not playing with a full deck
– Meshuggah
– Wacko
– Lights are on, but nobody's home

---

5   https://www.princeton.edu/~browning/snow.html. Accessed December 7, 2022.
6   Eskimo words for snow - Wikipedia. Accessed December 7, 2022.
7   QuickCheck: Do Eskimos have 100 words to describe snow? | The Star. Accessed December 7, 2022.

- *Has a screw loose*
- *Goofy*
- *Funny*
- *Bats in the belfry*
- *Nutty as a fruit cake*
- *Mad as a hatter*
- *Cuckoo*
- *Lost his marbles*
- *Went bananas*
- *Crackers*
- *Weird Out of his mind*
- *Not all there*
- *Odd*

WORDS WORDS WORDS

It is unfortunate that, in English, we can read the word disease as 'dis-ease', the lack of ease, which can be applied in the vernacular to mental problems. The medical use of the term 'disease', however, implies an underlying or causal biological dysfunction. Labelling a person with a mental problem as having a disease or as being diseased implies that there is something biologically awry with the person. This seems wrong and potentially perilous to do unless there is some sort of objective evidence of a biological abnormality, as interventions targeted on a biological abnormality may do no good and may cause harm, which might have disturbed Hippocrates.

We experience "different" people all the time. However, being different is not usually a marker of abnormal mental health, despite our visceral responses.

Why Some Problems are Illnesses; Others "Mental" Illnesses: The Challenge we Face

In everyday life, all of us experience mental health problems. They affect how people feel (sadness, depression or obsession), how they behave (fury, aggression, attention deficit disorder) and how they think (confusion, forgetfulness, fixation, aberrant thinking).

It is understandable that we have difficulty interpreting, explaining and reacting to mental health problems we see in ourselves and others. This is partly because there is widespread confusion about our understanding of the nature and biology of mental health. In this material we will attempt to clarify the understanding of what we know, what we are uncertain about and what we don't know about the nature, causes, meaning and treatment of mental health problems. Readers who understand the causes and meaning of mental health problems will understand the challenge of mental health labelling and diagnosis, the challenge of choosing the best treatments, and how our perception of mental health difficulties influences the interventions that clinicians recommend and that patients are willing to accept.

We All Influence Others

Virtually everyone – philosophers, psychiatrists, psychologists, politicians, dictators, propagandists, writers, news people, social scientists or just ordinary folks – tries to understand and influence the ways people think, feel and behave. We all have ways of influencing the people around us using common approaches. In fact, most changes in behavior, emotions and thinking are not caused by medical interventions but by our usual social interactions. However, medical professionals have the superpower of the pill. They are uniquely able to use a variety of pharmaceuticals that influence mental health.

It is worthwhile and informative to consider how mental problems differ from physical problems, like having a sore throat caused by a virus, having difficulty walking because of an injured knee or suffering pain from cancer.

In this material, we will use the terms 'mental illness' or 'mental disease' <u>only</u> when discussing mental health problems that a biological condition has definitely caused, like brain tumors, other neurological anomalies or endocrine abnormalities. On the other hand, we will use the terms 'mental dysfunction' or 'mental disorder' or 'mental health issue/problem' when there is, as far as medical science can determine at this time, <u>no identifiable biological cause,</u>

even if such a cause may eventually be discovered. In other words, we will take a conservative approach that does not automatically tag a person affected by mental health issues with having a biological/physiological abnormality – a medical label. When addressing both of these without differentiation, we will use the term 'mental (health) problem(s)'.

Definite brain abnormalities or another illness that affects the brain cause some mental problems. One example is hallucinations sometimes associated with a brain tumor. In addition, thyroid disease, Addison's disease and many other diseases of the body directly cause mental abnormalities; sometimes they do so indirectly through the burden they place on us. They often produce symptoms like depression, fatigue, anxiety, sleep disorders and, occasionally, aberrant thinking. It is also possible that abnormal brain development might lead to mental health issues[8]. In all these instances, the resulting symptoms are presentations of a true, identifiable illness – a biological abnormality – with a known cause. They have an identifiable physical cause, such as an injury, an infection,

maldevelopment of the components of the brain or an over- or under-production or utilization of substances that effect nerve function in the brain.

Very often, however, the brain might be normal, and the cause of mental health problems can be life circumstances like the death of a loved one, a devastating personal failure, having been sexually abused or having experienced bombing or shelling as a soldier or as 'collateral damage' (a hateful term!). These can give rise to a considerable level of mental dysfunction even though brain structure and function and the body's biology remain normal.[9]

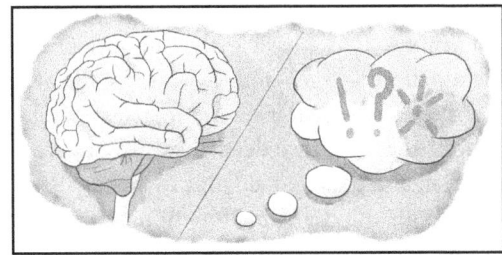

FIGURE 2.4.1: The Brain and the Mind

Mind vs Brain (FIGURE 2.4.1 illustrates these are different but not separate matters) ————————————

To understand the difference between a biological brain abnormality and environmentally caused mental dysfunction (a problem of the mind), we must recognize that the brain (a part of the body) and the mind (emerging from the action of the brain) – what thinks and feels and is our 'self' – are, to some extent distinct matters. A person's brain can be functioning correctly as brains go or it can be malfunctioning because of the effects of a disease

---

8   Neonatal abstinence syndrome is an example where the fetus might develop normally but display drug withdrawal symptoms because they have adapted to but are no longer exposed to a drug the mother was taking. Pogliani L, Schneider L, Dilillo D, Penagini F, Zuccotti GV. Paroxetine and neonatal withdrawal syndrome. BMJ Case Rep. 2010;2010: bcr12.2009.2528. Published 2010 Apr 29. doi:10.1136/bcr.12.2009.2528. https://www.ncbi.nlm.nih.gov/pmc/articles/PMC3047551/. Accessed December 7, 2022.

9   We discuss later that, although drugs influence thoughts, feelings and behavior in people, the drug's having effects does not imply a biologic abnormality existed. People become sleepy and relaxed when given Valium even though their biology was normal to begin with.

elsewhere in the body or an abnormality in the brain itself. Even with a correctly functioning brain, however, a person may have poor or confused ways of thinking (like serious biases or unfounded fears) or harbor inappropriate anger, fear or even violent feelings. Even a person with a brain or a mind that might be malfunctioning may have ways of thinking that correct for or work around those malfunctions. One example of the latter is the statement attributed – but not confirmed – to be from John Nash, the Nobel Laureate economist celebrated in the movie "A Beautiful Mind".[10] He often 'heard' voices but was purportedly eventually able to ignore these auditory hallucinations. It is possible that his brain was malfunctioning, generating what he 'heard', but it seems he used his mind to assert mental control that acknowledged those voices were not real, and that enabled him to ignore them. Clearly, his mind was malfunctioning because he experienced hallucinations, but his mind was also able to recognize the misperception. Consequently, he effectively prevented the hallucinations from having an adverse influence on his behavior or function.[11]

AN IMPORTANT RECOGNITION

We do not know for sure if people who experience hallucinations have a normal or malfunctioning brain or a normal or malfunctioning mind. At this point, we are simply ignorant, as science has not yet been able to determine which is the case. It is at least plausible that a malfunctioning brain can cause hallucinations (for example brain tumors or psychedelic drugs can interfere with brain function) or that a malfunctioning mind can. Regarding the latter, we all seem capable of having vivid and absorbing daydreams that can approximate hallucinating.

The 'Mind-Brain Dichotomy' is the distinction of the brain from the mind. People have spent lifetimes studying the mind-body problem without developing a universally accepted and persuasive conclusion. What is clear is that influencing our biology can change how we think, and that how we think influences how we feel. There is no absolute separation between the mind and the brain. Forming memories, having experiences and even thinking itself changes the structure of the brain – creating or altering new neural connections.

What is the Brain?

We can think of the brain in a simplified way as a collection of neurons. Neurons – nerve cells (there are other cells too) – have connections to other neurons through 'synapses' (inter-neuron cross-linkages), some of which are organized into 'circuits' – networks that connect parts of the brain together – that enable, to just name a few things, emotions, decision-making and control of the senses and limbs. There are about 85 billion (note the 'b') neurons with on the order of 100 trillion (that is 100,000 billion!) synapses. This is the 'hardware' – sometimes called 'wetware' – with which we think, feel and act. That is an incredibly large network, vastly greater than even the most sophisticated artificial intelligence 'neural network' that computer scientists have ever developed.

In addition to the network of neurons, there is a lot of chemistry in the brain. Substances like dopamine and serotonin play roles in how signals are conducted from neuron to neuron. It is this chemistry that many believe is influenced by psychoactive drugs that alter the way the brain works. However, evidence is lacking

---

10   https://www.imdb.com/title/tt0268978/. Accessed December 7, 2022.

11   https://abcnews.go.com/GMA/DrJohnson/story?id=126426&page=1#:~:text=Davis%20said%20Nash%20is%20an,consume%20him%2C%22%20Davis%20said.&text=In%20the%20movie%2C%20Nash%20sees,carries%20on%20conversations%20with%20them. Accessed December 7, 2022.

regarding specifics, like the effect of serotonin levels on depression.[12]

Perhaps it is useful to think about our brains thusly. Our genes construct the brain's neural network first – we inherit the basics – and the brain develops beyond that from our activities of learning, thinking, feeling, experiencing and doing. The chemistry of the brain also comes initially as an inheritance, but disease, our environment or those same activities can alter the brain's chemical environment. So can other factors.

Consider fear or anger, as examples. They can produce or be the result of chemical changes in the brain or in the body. Erotic fantasies can cause erotic excitement and familiar body changes. As another instance, hormones can cause our hearts to race when we are frightened, and a racing heart and running from danger might produce or be produced by thinking about or experiencing scary things. Usually, we are not able to distinguish if the flight led to feelings of fear, or the fear led to flight.

> One early theory of emotion, by William James, suggested that emotions occur because of a physiological reaction to events. When we see a lion, for example, he suggested we run and become fearful because we started to run. The more common opinion is that seeing a lion is frightening and causes the person to run. Is it the physiological response that causes the emotion, or the emotion that causes the physiological response? Does is make any practical difference?

Indeed, James' suggestion may be important mainly to philosophers; we won't delve into that here. However, the British National Health Service suggests that people who can "face their fears" by controlling breathing and avoiding flight are better able to cope and will feel less fearful.[13] Fear changes the body, the changes in the body can affect the chemistry of the brain, but we can use our minds – we can think – and exercise mental control to offset or moderate the effects of fearful situations. The thing to remember is that both the fearful reaction and the control of it likely result in subtle structural alterations in the brain and/or the chemicals that bathe it: it seems we constantly alter our brains!

The Rest of the Body and Brain Interact

So, the body/brain and the mind are integrated, inseparable. To understand the effect of the mind, consider that some people have a reaction of "blood-curdling" terror on seeing a snake or a spider. This might have been initiated by their Mom's reaction to these beasties, perhaps observed and experienced when they were children. The fear that Mom showed was palpable; it hit to the core and was the reaction of a very significant other. The fear stimulated 'fright and flight'-related hormones to be released in their own bodies. The brain remembers this. That reaction now happens every time they see an ambling arachnid or slithering serpent. Usually, there is no logical reason for the response (especially if that type of spider doesn't bite or the snake isn't poisonous), except for the mind causing and being affected by memories and chemical changes. However, some people can either damp-down or overcome their fear by thinking about it, or gradually approaching and withdrawing from the feared object[14] and eventually eliminating the response. Some even come to love the creepy-crawlies! Think of all the teenagers with pet tarantulas or boa constrictors. Some were

---

12 No evidence that depression is caused by low serotonin levels, finds comprehensive review -- ScienceDaily. Accessed December 7, 2022.

13 https://www.nhs.uk/conditions/stress-anxiety-depression/overcoming-fears/. From the National Health Service, Moodzone. Accessed January 31, 2019.

14 Smith, B.M., Smith, G.S. and Dymond, S. (2020), Relapse of anxiety-related fear and avoidance: Conceptual analysis of treatment with acceptance and commitment therapy. Jrnl Exper Analysis Behavior, 113: 87-104. https://onlinelibrary.wiley.com/doi/full/10.1002/jeab.573. Accessed December 7, 2022.

never conditioned to feel fear or, having been scared, they overcame it through mental effort. The point is that the whole person – mind and brain – dealt with the challenge and the mind won out.

When it comes to what we call 'mental health problems', both the mind and brain are holistically involved but the underlying cause of the problem can be rooted in either or both. Eventually we hope that neurological researchers and philosophers will develop a better understanding of brain events and how our context influences thinking and brain function.

We have a tendency to assume that all mental health problems have physical causes: diseases of the body – the brain in this case – true 'mental illnesses'. They don't!

We will address common mental problems later, but there is a serious matter that frustrates our healthcare system as it attempts to address them. That matter is that we have a tendency to assume that all mental health problems have physical causes: diseases of the body – the brain in this case – actual 'mental illnesses'. While it is true that some are caused by illnesses, many mental health problems are caused by dysfunctions in our minds – they are disorders of the mind – and considering them as physical diseases diverts care providers from effective interactive treatments – like psychotherapy and lifestyle changes – into the application of drugs that tend to impair the person's function or to cause harm.

We seem to consider that people who may be different or whom we perceive as different are somehow actually different, the victims of a physical problem (not unlike being infected with an STD) and we label and stigmatize them, in effect punishing them. Worse still, we often treat them with inappropriate drugs, and the drugs do cause them to change in some way. Mirabile dictu! They must have had something physically wrong with them!

But they didn't! As we have pointed out, those drugs would have had the same effect on most people. Those people were just different – upset, hurt, confused, the subjects of virtually any other deeply-felt human emotion, or they are just unique and unlike us.

What confounds things is that drugs do alter people's mental states, whether their biology is normal or abnormal. So, the drugs seem to be treating a physical illness, like antibiotics treat a bacterial infection. We all are aware that certain drugs affect everyone's mental state. For instance, lysergic acid diethylamide (LSD) causes some people to hallucinate. Diazepam (Valium) relaxes a person and can cause depression. Amphetamines ('uppers' in street-speak) can cause euphoria and might increase activity and anxiety. These drug effects occur whether or not people have abnormal biology. They do affect the brain, but they are not correcting a brain problem. There was likely nothing wrong with the brain… however, one might wonder if there was something wrong with the mind – the thinking and decision-making – of the person who elected to accept the prescription!

We should note that there is a great deal of research underway into finding apparent causes – particularly genetic and developmental origins – of mental health problems, especially major ones, such as severe autism, psychosis and schizophrenia. Stay tuned, as this may be a long-time unfolding. But for now, the biological causes of many mental health problems remain a mystery.

Drugs as Possible Treatments for Mental Health Problems

Drugs can, themselves, cause – as well as allay or moderate – mental problems. They can have a powerful influence on mental health. Consequently, medical schools include Psychiatry in their curricula because physicians are the one group of care providers that in most jurisdictions are authorized to prescribe drugs. Other than drugs, physicians and non-physician mental health workers all use the same tools as the rest of us to address mental health issues.

A big fly in the ointment is the professionals' flight to a physical cause, a physical illness that is an expression of abnormal biology. That is not a minor matter! The belief that most problems of the mind are problems of the body predisposes diagnosticians to search, first, for pharmaceutical solutions. This is true of many psychiatrists who argue that there are no important differences between problems labelled 'illness' and those labelled 'mental illness'.[15] They see only 'brain problems'. Consequently, they often recommend medical and pharmaceutical solutions rather than other less intrusive and effective non-medicinal maneuvers. This is why we distinguish mental illness as a disease from mental dysfunction.

This equating of mental problems with illness is common despite our recognition that abnormal biology is not a necessary condition for mental health problems and that pharmaceuticals are often not the most appropriate intervention.[16] We will, later, discuss the role of exercise and of verbal psychotherapy (talk therapy), where therapists work with patients with the objective of identifying issues that disturb their mental state and then help patients to take steps to moderate or overcome them. In a sense, this is helping patients to 'heal' themselves. It is interesting to note that researchers assert that verbal therapies apparently affect the brain itself, causing or strengthening linkages between neurons. Therefore,

another point is that drugs are not the only interventions that affect the brain directly.[17]

Drugs Versus Placebos

We should note that many clinical trials of psychoactive drugs have a high placebo-response rate, meaning that patients respond similarly to placebos as to active drugs. In controlled trials of medication for major depression, for instance, more patients benefit without active medication if both the active drug group and the placebo group are equally able to have more interactions with counsellors. Indeed, with intensive counselling it may be difficult to demonstrate that psychoactive pharmaceuticals are more effective than a placebo combined with counselling is.[18] Kandel has stated that *"Imaging has even predicted, in some cases of depression, which patients are best treated with drugs, with psychotherapy, or with both."* [19] However, no one in the clinical world reports using brain imaging to decide who should receive drugs.

RECOGNITION OF DISSENSION

Others have challenged Kandel's assertion, indicating that no one has yet been able to use imaging or any other test to demonstrate scientifically that we can predict which patients will respond to psychotherapy alone, to drugs alone or to both. Perhaps in the future, based on large collections of data, the dream of using objective biomarkers to predict who is most likely to benefit or be harmed by treatments will be realized. However, we are not there yet.

Furthermore, retrospective studies that show differences in the brains of people labelled mentally

---

15   Kendell, R.E. The distinction between mental and physical illness. DOI: 10.1192/bjp.178.6.490 Published 1 June 2001. http://bjp.rcpsych.org/content/178/6/490. Accessed December 7, 2022.

16   Roose SP, Rutherford BR, Wall MM, Thase ME. Practising evidence-based medicine in an era of high placebo response: number needed to treat reconsidered. *Br J Psychiatry*. 2016;208(5):416-20. https://www.ncbi.nlm.nih.gov/pmc/articles/PMC4853640/. Accessed December 7, 2022.

17   The Disordered Mind, 2018, E.R. Kandel, pg. 105.

18   Roose SP, Rutherford BR, Wall MM, Thase ME. Practising evidence-based medicine in an era of high placebo response: number needed to treat reconsidered. *Br J Psychiatry*. 2016;208(5):416-20. https://www.ncbi.nlm.nih.gov/pmc/articles/PMC4853640/. Accessed December 7, 2022.

19   ibidem: Kandel, pg 105-106.

ill who were treated with drugs, versus those not labelled mentally ill, do not necessarily support the idea that brain dysfunction was responsible for the initial problem. This is because drug treatment might be the only reason the brains appear different. A key aspiration of mental health researchers is to be able to use objective markers, including brain imaging, to distinguish people who have mental health problems from those who appear to be mentally healthy. Time will tell if this is possible.

Life is Rough on the Mind

In Dickens' novel 'Oliver Twist', two children who had no biological abnormalities, at least as identified by the author, learned to behave in peculiar ways when one of the characters taught them to steal. Abnormal biology just does not explain all mental problems…or perhaps even many of them. We are all immersed in a somewhat toxic stew called 'life'! And life, like an election, "has consequences", many of them mental!

How We Think About Problems Affects How We Treat Them

How people think about problems determines or at least influences the solutions they consider. Everyone who wants to support improvements in mental health and in mental health services must understand the differences between problems merely <u>labelled</u> an 'illness' and those actually a product of an illness. This is of more than academic interest because

adherents to the illness model are inclined to use medication as a first choice, despite little or no evidence of a biological problem for which medication might be the most effective solution.[20]

This is why many experts reject the 'illness' interpretation of mental health problems[21] [22] [23]. It portrays the sufferer as a victim of a biological malady, unable to help her or himself without medication or a physician's intervention. They prefer another model, where safe non-medicinal interventions are at least the first choice, unless the person proves to have a biological (brain-based or body-based) abnormality or is in unmanageable distress, out of control, an immediate danger to self or other, or when other non-medicinal maneuvers have failed to provide a remedy.

Another point is that, in the absence of cure for the speculated mental illness, care takers can enrol the person in a lifetime of symptomatic, not curative, treatment. Proponents of mental health drugs don't claim they are a cure in the same way as antibiotics cure infections.

We do not wish to detract from or demean the efforts of those investigators seeking biological causes for mental health problems. If there are such causes, we want to know about them and deal directly with them. If, for example, genetic abnormalities underlie some mental health problems, we must know about that and determine if there are any interventions or strategies to prevent or ameliorate the effects of that abnormality. But we cannot just assume a biological cause. Phenylketonuria[24]

20 Cipriani, A., Geddes, J.R. Placebo for depression: we need to improve the quality of scientific information but also reject too simplistic approaches or ideological nihilism, BMC Med. 2014; 12: 105. Published online 2014 Jun 25. doi: 10.1186/1741-7015-12-105. http://www.ncbi.nlm.nih.gov/pmc/articles/PMC4070084/. Accessed December 7, 2022.

21 Plato Not Prozac. New York: HarperCollins, 1999. Accessed December 7, 2022.

22 Kinderman, P., Why we need to abandon disease model of mental health care scientific American blog http://blogs.scientificamerican.com/mind-guest-blog/why-we-need-to-abandon-the-disease-model-of-mental-health-care/November 17, 2014. http://blogs.scientificamerican.com/mind-guest-blog/why-we-need-to-abandon-the-disease-model-of-mental-health-care/. Accessed December 7, 2022.

23 Peter Kinderman, A Prescription for Psychiatry. (September 2014) Palgrave Macmillan. Accessed 13 August 2015.

24 US National Library of Medicine, Genetics Home Reference, Your Guide to Understanding Genetic Conditions. https://ghr.nlm.nih.gov/condition/phenylketonuria. Accessed December 7, 2022.

is an example we have mentioned elsewhere of a genetic condition producing mental disturbances, including retardation, where the biochemistry of the problem is well known, and where the simple solution follows from our understanding of the problem.

Defining and Remediating Mental Health Problems

The suffering from mental health dysfunction is as real and commonplace and often as important as the suffering from biological illness. Consequently, it is equally important to discover the cause or origin of such problems and to apply safe and effective remedies. This is particularly relevant because most drugs produce not only their desired effects, but also undesirable adverse reactions. Many antidepressants, for example, are associated with changes in libido, weight gain and, consequentially, decreased energy and activity.

We might also mention that mental health problems can be 'infectious'; they are communicable. People are familiar with terms like "infectious enthusiasm". When someone behaves in even a mildly deranged way, including signalling depression or showing profound upset, this often influences the mood of the people around them, even though it doesn't change their biology.

Jumping directly to drug intervention when dealing with behavioral problems is especially concerning. The reaction to and acceptability of behaviors is not societally uniform. Most would accept that people in different cultures may think, feel and behave differently, even though they share a common biology. However, acceptable behavior in Manhattan might not be acceptable in Smallville. Similarly, one household or social cluster may regard a behavior as okay, but another might frown on it. Some communities welcome strangers while others are xenophobic. Context affects the acceptability of behaviors. The nature of individuals influences things as well. One teacher

may enjoy working with an active, curious and assertive child. However, another teacher might interpret the same behavior as a sign of an attention deficit disorder (ADD – a psychiatric label). Sometimes, clinicians cannot determine if a child is hyperactive or if it's just that the parents and teachers are underactive.

In other words, the thoughts and behaviors associated with mental health problems engender different reactions according to culture, geographic location, school, household and observers' biases and perceptions. Behavior regarded as normal by some, others can consider as a sign of mental illness or criminality. In North America, two people might commit the same type of crime. Depending on the attitude of the local community and local clinicians, one might be sent to prison; the other, to a mental hospital.

So, why, again, do people use the terms 'mental disorder' or 'mental dysfunction' to describe some patients with certain problems but use the term 'mental illness' to describe others who have the same behaviors, urges or complaints? For example, some may consider depressed feelings and low energy as signs and symptoms of a life problem or decreased physical fitness, something that has affected the mind. Others' may consider people with those same problems as having a 'mental illness', implying a physical brain problem. Could it be that they consider it thusly because they believe they can intervene with a 'simple' drug rather than investing time and energy in human-human interaction or a lifestyle change to intervene on the latter? Are they just lazy or too busy?

Purpose of Mental Health Care is to Change Thoughts, Feelings and Behavior

On the face of it, Psychiatry seems complex because few people, including physicians and psychiatrists, can give concise and clear definitions to the problems people have, to the purposes of mental health care or to the objective measures of the success of treatment.

Mental health interventions are similar to other health interventions because their goals are to improve comfort, function and lifespan. Mental health interventions are different, though, in that they aim to achieve the goals of health care indirectly by helping change how people think, what they feel and how they behave.

The Canadian Mental Health Association declares, "*Mental illness... results in the significant impairment of an individual's cognitive [thinking], affective [feeling] or relational [behavior] abilities*"[25] [our insertions]. This does not mean that anyone who feels poorly, has aberrant or confused thinking or behaves abnormally has a physical illness or biological dysfunction. As we mentioned, the use of the term 'illness' is a problem.

Some people seem to believe that mental health workers are endowed with special powers, different from those of ordinary physicians or the rest of us. It's as if they command esoteric knowledge, mystic skills, exceptional talents or sophisticated tools to address mental health problems. They don't! It may be that they have more experience and familiarity with people's mental problems and may have a sensitive and disciplined approach to them because of the focus of their practices. However, except for being able to prescribe, all of us use similar ways of recognizing problems and using interventions (examples follow later) to influence people around us. The activities of relatives, friends, acquaintances, teachers – everybody – not just those of physicians, psychiatrists, psychologists and mental health workers – affect the people they meet. Sometimes this influence is deliberate. At other times our influence is accidental or unintended.

We reinforce the fact that both people with normal biology as well as those with biochemical or physiological brain abnormalities, all respond to psychotropic drugs. Almost everyone who takes amphetamines feels more energetic and becomes more active. Almost everyone who takes diazepam (e.g., Valium [TR]) feels more relaxed and becomes less active. The effect a drug has does not necessarily illuminate the cause of a problem.

We try to understand mental health[26] by considering what people have learned and how they think, their cultural and social context – where, how and with whom they live – and what we know of their medical or drug-taking history. It is worth reiterating that thinking about mental health mainly as a product of learning and life context leads to non-pharmaceutical solutions, while emphasizing the physiology and biochemistry of behavior leads almost inevitably to medical treatments, with their potential harm. Non-pharmaceutical interventions for mental health problems, including life-style changes and counselling, are often successful and rarely detrimental. Sometimes, people may need drugs and the drugs may help, but they do put some people at risk of adverse drug reactions.

Researchers appear to be making progress towards understanding the workings of the brain and, therefore, learning why and how people function in normal or abnormal ways. Others claim to understand behavior by examining how our parents and significant others behaved and how they affected us as children. Behavioral psychologists have developed and tested effective techniques that successfully

---

25 Canadian Mental Health Association, Workplace Mental Health Promotion: A How To Guide. https://cmha-east. on.ca/index.php/en/workplace-mental-health-promotion. Accessed December 7, 2022.

26 The only purposes of mental health interventions are to change thoughts feelings and behavior. For convenience, the word behavior may be used to include not only behavior that also thoughts and feelings.

alter thoughts, feelings and behavior.[27] [28] Psychiatrists, therefore, are not alone in claiming that they really understand why people decide, feel, and do things.

It may be that efforts to understand brain activity by analyzing medical images and electrical signals or using biochemical tests will prove to be fruitful and provide meaningful explanations of how the mind works. We must consider this critically, however, to ensure that we are not adopting a pseudoscience, more related to phrenology[29] than medical science. We must evaluate the evidence.

A FEW WORDS ABOUT PHRENOLOGY

Phrenology, an ancient, debunked pseudoscience, was based on the notion that the size and activity of our brains influence the size and shape of our skulls. That seemed to make sense long ago but was not based on actual measurement of the brain-skull congruence. According to phrenologists, accurate measures of the lumps and bumps on peoples' skulls were useful in assessments of their character and personality. We wonder if having a lump acquired in a high school fight might be indicative of one's genius. What do you think? Many experts believe that more sophisticated imaging and medical testing might eventually uncover the truth.

Seeing the Brain Functioning ———

It is important that we recognize that a great deal of research is underway in applying functional Magnetic Resonance Imaging (fMRI)[30] and other advanced forms of imaging to measuring at least some (mostly at a gross level) aspects of brain function. As an example, one can use fMRI to see changes in brain blood flow that researchers consider is indicative of a specific part of the brain's becoming active, such as during the decision-making process.[31] Investigators describe that areas of the brain 'light up' in the resulting images, indicating they are active, and they do so in identifiable sequences. Researchers believe the sequences show which brain 'circuits', or connected areas of the brain, enable our brains to do complicated things like make decisions.

Researchers have been making serious efforts to identify structural changes that might explain abnormal mental health and claim to have identified changes in the brains of some people with mental health disorders. However, it is not clear whether the changes in brain images reflect an underlying problem or are changes related to the use of the psychotropic drugs.[32]

With another method, PET (Positron Emission Tomography) imaging,[33] one can see increases in the brain's metabolism of

---

27   https://us.sagepub.com/en-us/nam/journal/psychological science#description. Accessed December 7, 2022.

28   Journal of the Experimental Analysis of Behavior. https://journals.sagepub.com/home/pss. Accessed December 7, 2022.

29   Phrenologists believed that behavior could be understood and predicted by examining the shape of the skull. Some psychiatrists believe that behavior can be understood by examining images of the brain or the chemicals in your brain. Of course, no one has yet been able to take a picture of a brain or analyze the chemicals in the brain to determine what you are thinking now or how you are likely to behave in the future.

30   Overview of Functional Magnetic Resonance Imaging, Gary H. Glover Neurosurg Clin N Am, 2011 Apr; 22(2): 133–139.   doi: 10.1016/j.nec.2010.11.001.   https://www.ncbi.nlm.nih.gov/pmc/articles/PMC3073717/. Accessed December 7, 2022.

31   https://www.psychologytoday.com/blog/think-act-be/201605/using-brain-scans-diagnose-mental-disorders. Accessed December 7, 2022.

32   "It is well established that the drugs used to treat a mental disorder, for example, may induce long-lasting biochemical and even structural changes [including in the brain], which in the past were claimed to be the cause of the disorder, but may actually be an effect of the treatment." E. Valenstein, Blaming the Brain: www.cchr.org. http://www.cchr.org/quick-facts/no-brain-scans-for-mental-illness.html. Accessed December 7, 2022.

33   Positron emission tomography for brain research Masahiro Mishina J Nippon Med Sch. 2008 Apr;75(2):68-76. doi: 10.1272/jnms.75.68. https://pubmed.ncbi.nlm.nih.gov/18475026/. Accessed December 7, 2022.

glucose (sugar), which also appears to be associated with the parts of the brain becoming active during a cognitive (thinking) or motor (motion-affecting) process. This has helped scientists to conjecture about brain function while the brain undertakes the steps involved in a thought process and helps identify the areas involved and the sequence of functions the brain performs.

There are limits, though. Some researchers have attempted to use this technology to recognize if a person is telling the truth or lying. So far, the courts do not consider the results of these tests as evidence. The fact is that, at least so far, examining brain images cannot reliably tell us if the person is telling the truth or lying or looking out the window and seeing farm animals or just imagining them. We certainly cannot yet use these images to tell <u>what</u> a person is thinking or <u>how</u> they are feeling. In some sense, what the images show is kind of 'tracer' of brain function, much like we might trace some biochemical process in the intestines or how the liver processes glucose. Maybe someday these or more advanced techniques may enable us to understand the process of dysfunctional thinking or the generation of hallucinations in our brains. For now, these

techniques are blunt ones and the science associated with them is relatively immature.

Neither phrenologists nor modern MRI/fMRI/PET experts – and certainly not psychiatrists or psychologists using brain imaging or any other technique – can interpret people's thoughts, assess their characters, predict if they are likely to be kind or violent, determine whether or not they are a logical and coherent thinker or determine that they qualify for a mental illness label.[34] [35] [36] Brain imaging techniques and blood tests cannot even distinguish people who are happy from those who are sad! There is some early suggestion, however, that brain imaging may eventually help us to begin to understand the brains of persons with selected mental problems, such as autism[37] and schizophrenia[38].

On the other hand, independent, objective blood tests and diagnostic images can identify people who have certain cancers or hormonal abnormalities that are known to influence mental health. The presence of exceptionally high- or low-levels of thyroid hormone marks people as having thyroid disease, and an x-ray image is often sufficient to diagnose cancer. It is important to recognize that these are medical

34 https://www.psychologytoday.com/blog/think-act-be/201605/using-brain-scans-diagnose-mental-disorders. Accessed December 7, 2022.

35 Accessed December 7, 2022. "It is well established that the drugs used to treat a mental disorder, for example, may induce long-lasting biochemical and even structural changes [including in the brain], which in the past were claimed to be the cause of the disorder, but may actually be an effect of the treatment." —Dr. Elliot Valenstein, biopsychologist, author, Blaming the Brain".
No Brain Scans for Mental Illness: www.cchr.org: What do brain scans show? Find out the truth about the technique used by psychiatry to supposedly show mental illness. Learn about yet another scam used by these pseudo scientists to justify their "profession." Read the facts from the Citizen's Commission on Human Rights. http://www.cchr.org/quick-facts/no-brain-scans-for-mental-illness.html. Accessed December 7, 2022.

36 http://www.nytimes.com/2005/10/18/health/psychology/can-brain-scans-see-depression.html?_r=0. Accessed December 7, 2022.

37 A systematic review and meta-analysis of the fMRI investigation of autism spectrum disorders. Philipa RCM, Dauvermanna MR, Whalleya HC, Baynhama K, Lawriea SM, Stanfield AC. Neuroscience & Biobehavioral Reviews Vol 36, Issue 2, Feb 2012, pgs 901-942. https://www.sciencedirect.com/science/article/abs/pii/S0149763411002016?via%3Dihub. Accessed December 7, 2022.

38 Brain structure, function, and neurochemistry in schizophrenia and bipolar disorder—a systematic review of the magnetic resonance neuroimaging literature. Birur B, Kraguljac NV, Shelton NPJ, Schizophr RC, et al. 3, 15 (2017). https://doi.org/10.1038/s41537-017-0013-9. Accessed December 7, 2022.

conditions that clearly influence thoughts, mood and behavior.[39]

This is the key message: there are, as yet few or no objective and reliable biomarkers that identify people, absent a biological disease that affects the function of the brain, who should have the 'mental illness' label. Right now, that is always a subjective clinical judgement. And diagnosing an 'illness' should not be based on a subjective clinical judgement.

Summary

When there is direct evidence of a biological abnormality causing mood or behavioral disturbance, we consider the person as having a mental illness. In this case, the cause of this illness does not originate in the mind, despite the effects the illness may have on the mind. The cause is either a biological abnormality in the body (again, a good example is Addison's Disease) that affects the brain or a biological abnormality in the brain (a brain tumor or an anatomical or physiological brain abnormality), either of which may affect the mind.

Unfortunately, even when there are no objective signs of abnormal biology, some diagnosticians may label the problem an illness, a mental illness and sometimes speculate – intellectually, they 'reverse engineer' – that there is an underlying, yet undiscovered, biological abnormality. But that is just speculation! The doctor is applying the term 'illness' improperly. In this instance, the phrase 'mentally ill' is a mislabel; it is not an attribute of the patient. This is not intended to demean the importance of the problem and it does not preclude the use of drugs in seeking to change the person's mental state.

The absence of objective signs that explain the patient's condition is characteristic of much mental dysfunction. Applying the term 'mental illness' is akin to labelling a problem 'Idiopathic', which, while sounding impressive, means we don't know what the cause is (you can read about this in the chapter on Etiologies). Similarly, the term 'epistaxis' used to describe a nosebleed is not an explanation of why the nose is bleeding. As of now, there are no or only vague or conjectural biomarkers of mental dysfunction.

If people are having mental health problems and they have the biomarkers of a physical disease or dysfunction, we should really regard them as 'ill', not 'mentally ill'. We should indicate that they have a disorder in thinking, feeling or behavior that is a symptom caused by an underlying disease. Someone with a brain tumor, who is experiencing hallucinations, has an illness (a brain tumor) and has an associated mental dysfunction, disorder or problem. Similarly, a person with abnormal brain structure (examples being abnormal neural communication among the parts of the brain, a brain injury damaging a part of the brain, or an abnormality in brain biochemistry) also has an illness. Regretfully, as we have mentioned, some speculate that abnormal behavior and mood is always a reflection of an underlying biological brain abnormality. This is like branding a person a suicide who accidently fell off a building and died.

We all know that normal people can learn to behave in abnormal ways. Parents may teach or otherwise condition children to behave badly. Often the moods of sadness and anger reflect the context a person lives in, rather than being a sign of abnormal biology. Sadness and anger are unpleasant, but they are part and parcel of life, particularly social life.

It may avail that some day we will be able to measure and objectively interpret brain activity, analyze bodily fluids or identify defective genes to learn what we are thinking, why we are thinking in a certain way and whether or not a person has a mental illness or a propensity to mental disorders like violent behavior. In 2023, however, we are not there, and we very

---

39 People with low levels of thyroid hormone have less energy, sometimes interpreted as feeling depressed; people with brain tumors are more likely to suffer from hallucinations and thinking problems.

much doubt we will be there in the foresee-
able future. The tools we have do not enable
anyone to use objective biological markers to
diagnose or predict thinking or even flagrant
mental abnormalities.[40]

---

40   This is exemplified by people who go out and harm themselves or others after seeing a mental health professional
     who had no apprehension whatever that such a dire event might follow.

Chapter 5: ——— Thinking About Mental Health Problems

KEYWORDS: Understanding Mental Health Problems, Describing Mental Health Problems, Mental Health Labels, Lifestyle Changes, Placebo Response

ABSTRACT: People labelled with mental health problems fall into one of five categories (and those in category 5 should not be so labelled!). One group includes people who have biological problems that can cause mental problems, for example brain tumors or thyroid disease, which are relatively easy to diagnose. Another group comprises people who have biological problems that are more difficult to diagnose. These people often suffer for a long time because professionals ascribe a "mental illness" as the cause of their problem. The third group, perhaps the largest, consists of people who have mental health problems where the cause is not known. People in this group might have a medical condition that researchers have not yet discovered or they may have suffered from issues in their life contexts that no one has recognized. The fourth group includes people whose lives are complex and dysfunctional, perhaps because of a poor education or growing up in an abusive household. And finally, the fifth group consists of people (mis)labelled as having mental health problems merely because they are different from other people in the community. These latter folks might feel comfortable with themselves, and often make meaningful, not harmful, contributions to society. However, those around them, even sometimes clinicians, feel the need to attribute a 'mental' label. One example may be some of those labelled as having "Autistic Spectrum Disorder", a label that has been retroactively pinned on some Nobel Laurate scientists.

Introduction

Feeling confused, deep down in the dumps, over-excited, intensely lonely, furious, unloved, scared or upset seem to be the essence of life itself! We all have these feelings. Sometimes, though, they can over-power us and interfere with our ability to get on with our lives. Sometimes they can even sicken us. Many are common problems, albeit mental health problems. Especially if they compromise our cognition, emotions or actions, they can drive us to visit a clinician.

A Framework for Thinking About the Treatment of Mental Problems

Mental health problems are an important and common[41] part of medical practice. Yet many clinicians are uncomfortable dealing with them.[42] Successful mental health interventions help people to feel better, to think more coherently, and to act in ways the person and community feel are more appropriate and worthwhile. We must be aware, though, that inappropriate interventions may harm us or those around us. Most of us have had hurt feelings from mistaken words, even when the speaker has good intentions.

Unfortunately, we often have a limited understanding of mental health problems. As we have pointed out, many people diagnosed with mental illness do not demonstrate objective evidence of abnormal biology or of any "biochemical imbalance" (whatever that is).

Fortunately, there are many effective interventions that enable clinicians to help improve a person's mental health. These include, but are not limited to, verbal discussions, counselling regarding relationships, rewards and punishments, suggestions for lifestyle modifications, and pharmaceuticals. Prescribing the latter is the unique role of physicians. Unfortunately, despite the risk of harmful effects, clinicians often overprescribe psychoactive drugs[43] and they are abused by people who buy street drugs and self-medicate.

In the case of serious or extreme problems, both experts and non-experts rarely disagree that there are people who need medical help.

However, clinicians usually want to make a diagnosis – to determine the cause of a problem – before they prescribe or otherwise intervene. This is because accurate diagnosis and understanding of the problem should determine the choice of appropriate treatment. The ideal circumstance is that clinicians understand the physiology and epidemiology of a disease or dysfunction and have precise information about which and how often medications or other interventions will help or harm. Failure to determine the cause of a problem means that some people with a health problem will receive treatment that is of unknown effectiveness and that might cause further problems. This has important implications for those with mental health issues because the causes for these problems are often elusive.

Unfortunately, there are many controversies regarding if and why a person is mentally dysfunctional, i.e., to figure out what is wrong.

Pinning psychiatric labels on patients with mental health problems using DSM (the Diagnosis and Statistical Manual of Mental Disorders used in Psychiatry) criteria is sometimes contentious and often unreliable[44]. A diagnostic label that describes the problem (for example saying a person who feels depressed has the diagnosis 'Depression') does not add to our understanding of why the person feels depressed, nor does it provide a clear indication of what to do about it. Without clear, objectively measurable and well-differentiated criteria, determining a cause for a person's problem is a blind search in the dark. This difficulty that

41 Canadian Mental Health Association, Fast Facts About Mental Illness. https://cmha.ca/brochure/fast-facts-about-mental-illness/. Accessed December 7, 2022.

42 Ross LE, Vigod S, Wishart J, et al. Barriers and facilitators to primary care for people with mental health and/or substance use issues: a qualitative study. BMC Fam Pract. 2015; 16:135. Published 2015 Oct 13. doi:10.1186/s12875-015-0353-3. https://www.ncbi.nlm.nih.gov/pmc/articles/PMC4604001/. Accessed December 7, 2022.

43 Fournier JC, DeRubeis RJ, Hollon SD, et al. Antidepressant drug effects and depression severity: a patient-level meta-analysis. JAMA. 2010;303(1):47–53. doi:10.1001/jama.2009.1943. https://www.ncbi.nlm.nih.gov/pmc/articles/PMC3712503/. Accessed December 7, 2022.

44 Davis KA, Sudlow CL, Hotopf M. Can mental health diagnoses in administrative data be used for research? A systematic review of the accuracy of routinely collected diagnoses. BMC Psychiatry. 2016;16: 263. Published 2016 Jul 26. doi:10.1186/s12888-016-0963-x. https://www.ncbi.nlm.nih.gov/pmc/articles/PMC4960739/. Accessed December 7, 2022.

everyone has in categorizing mental problems makes it challenging to determine how best to intervene. Later chapters discuss issues related to measuring, labeling and treating mental health problems.

We believe it is worthwhile to think systematically about the diagnosis of mental health problems. We propose to do this by considering a relatively simple framework for categorizing patients. We provide here a kind of meta-diagnostic process for application before proceeding with the classical diagnostic method. This framework incorporates a five-step scheme that defines our approach to the diagnosis of mental health problems. The framework we proffer encourages the consideration of the knowledge of the biology and circumstantial origins of mental health abnormalities for each individual patient.

We will present the framework and illustrate it by visualizing a journey towards intervention as a walk, with a shopping cart, through the interconnected rooms of the **Mental Health Diagnosis Emporium**. See FIGURE 2.5.1.

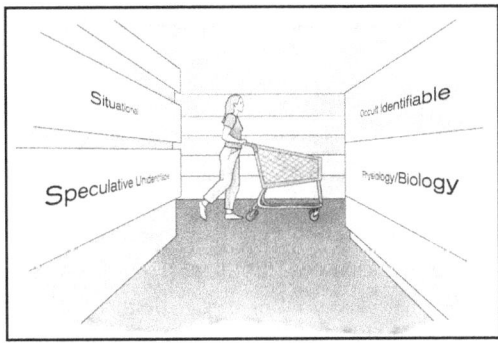

FIGURE 2.5.1: The Mental Health Diagnosis Emporium

The Framework: Shopping for a Diagnosis or Explanation of Mental Health Problems

We start our shopping expedition by entering the Diagnosis Emporium's **Room 1 – The Room of Identifiable Physiological/ Biological Causes** that may have effects on mental health.[45] This room has shelves full of many common, known, diagnosable biological illnesses. The room exists because some people have mental health problems that a known biological illness clearly caused and the clinician can and must identify and treat it.

We mentioned before that patients with thyroid disease might experience anxiety, depression, mania, fatigue, emotional lability, insomnia and irritability. There is some suggestion that thyroid abnormalities might even present as schizophrenic thought disorder.[46] Brain tumors and identifiable brain pathology (like a developmental abnormality or an injury of the brain) may also present with thought disorders including visual and auditory hallucinations.[47]

If the correct diagnosis is in stock in Room 1, we select it, put it in our shopping cart, leave the store and treat the underlying disease that is causing the problem. The treatment of mental health problems caused by medical diseases with objective biomarkers is the treatment of the underlying condition, perhaps with appropriate support for the patient's residual psychosocial issues.

Ok, what If we can't find a diagnosis in Room 1?

Then we proceed through the door on the far wall to **Room 2 – The Room of Occult Identifiable Causes**. This room has no

45 Welch KA, Carson AJ. When psychiatric symptoms reflect medical conditions. Clin Med (Lond). 2018 Feb;18(1):80-87. doi: 10.7861/clinmedicine.18-1-80. PMID: 29436444; PMCID: PMC6330910. https://www.ncbi.nlm.nih.gov/pmc/articles/PMC6330910/ . Accessed Jan 15, 2024.

46 Santos NC, Costa P, Ruano D, et al. Revisiting thyroid hormones in schizophrenia. J Thyroid Res. 2012; 2012:569147. https://www.ncbi.nlm.nih.gov/pmc/articles/PMC3321576/. Accessed December 7, 2022.

47 Teeple RC, Caplan JP, Stern TA. Visual hallucinations: differential diagnosis and treatment. Prim Care Companion J Clin Psychiatry. 2009;11(1):26-32. https://www.ncbi.nlm.nih.gov/pmc/articles/PMC2660156/. Accessed December 7, 2022.

lighting; finding what we need will require a diligent and time-consuming search in the dark. This room holds the less-common diagnoses of people with mental health problems who have identifiable medical conditions, with biomarkers, but that their doctor has not yet considered, searched for or diagnosed. We search diligently but must be aware that, occasionally, obscure diagnoses will remain undiscovered for a long time. When the clinician and patient tire of searching or cannot think of possible diagnoses and solutions, they must consider that the problem may reside in rooms 3 or 4. The room we are in, Room 2, connects to rooms that address problems having no biological abnormality or at least none that anyone has yet discovered. We will go there soon.

Many rare conditions that produce disturbed mental health are, conceptually, in a space like Room 2. Some might take years of investigation to discover and formulate as a diagnosis. Clinicians often label patients having these rare but diagnosable and treatable conditions with a 'mental illness' diagnosis despite having an addressable biological disease that the clinician had not yet considered.[48] Until a rare diagnosis has been made and confirmed, there is just no way to know for sure whether the person's problem is in Room 2 or is elsewhere in the store. It is possible or even likely that treating people in this group with illness-correcting interventions like pharmaceuticals will be a mistake. Sometimes the intervention may appear to 'correct' the 'underlying problem' but that may be an illusion, as they would have affected everyone that way. At other times they may make the problem worse. It may help to realize that there are often many causes of a problem and that finding which one

is correct is not easy. For instance, the website RIGHTDIAGNOSIS™ listed 3,235 causes of fatigue.[49] Most doctors do not wade through all these possibilities or they stop looking after considering only a small fraction. This means they might decamp and just label some of the rare causes of persistent fatigue as 'depression' (a symptom, not a cause), thereby assigning a mental health or psychosomatic label to patients who have uncommon but potentially identifiable medical problems.[50]

A DIAGNOSIS IN ROOM 2

The book, "The Medical Detectives", describes a woman who endured years of being diagnosed with a psychiatric problem, being treated with powerful psychoactive drugs, having shock treatments (ECT: Electro-Convulsive Therapy) and spending weeks in psychiatric hospitals. An inquisitive physician and an ophthalmologist, on noticing something about her appearance, eventually determined that she had Wilson's Disease, a problem with her metabolism of Copper. After successful treatment, her psychiatric symptoms abated, and she recovered with only mild tremors. (The Medical Detectives, Berton Roueche, Truman Talley Books/Plume, pp. 345-360, 1991)

To help and to avoid harming people with one of these rare causes, clinicians must take a systematic – and possibly long-term – approach to diagnosis. This usually means stepwise excluding the rare conditions that produce mental health abnormalities. Using a checklist of the latter might help the physician. Medications or other interventions may provide symptomatic help, in the interim.

Meanwhile, if we discover that the cause for the patient's problem is there in Room 2, we pick it up from the shelf, put it in our cart and

48 Rare Disease U.K., The National Alliance for people with rare diseases & all who support them also cited in reference 8 above- It's Not All in My Head. http://www.raredisease.org.uk/media/1588/the-rare-reality-an-insight-into-the-patient-and-family-experience-of-rare-disease.pdf. Accessed December 7, 2022.

49 RIGHTDIAGNOSIS https://www.rightdiagnosis.com/sym/fatigue.htm. Accessed November 10, 2018.

50 "It's not all in my head!" - The complex relationship between rare diseases and mental health problems. Orphanet J Rare Dis. 2017;12(1):29. Published 2017 Feb 27. doi:10.1186/s13023-017-0591-7. https://www.icd10data.com/ICD10CM/Codes/F01-F99/F30-F39/F32-/F32.0. Accessed December 7, 2022.

leave the Emporium. We have what we needed! Now we must treat that cause.

Suppose, however, we didn't luck out in Room 2. Then, we can proceed to the far wall and through the door into **Room 3 – The Room of Speculative and Unidentifiable Causes**. Even though the lights are on in this room, there is nothing in it other than clouds of smoke, fun-house mirrors and ghostly illusions. Our advice is to keep going, leaving all that is here as it lies. This room contains the speculative diagnoses of people with mental health problems applied by doctors lacking objective evidence of the cause's being a biological abnormality but give it a putative biological name. It may, in fact, be that the patient has a biological abnormality that researchers have not yet identified, but there are no tests, at least yet, to identify what it is. An untestable diagnosis is mere speculation! It is akin to saying a problem is due to miasma (bad air) or phlogiston (a fire-like element hypothesized by alchemists).

In these cases, clinicians, biased by an unfounded belief in a hypothetical biological disturbance – a phantasm – sometimes prescribe drugs. The presenting problems for these people are abnormalities in how they think, feel and behave, which physicians believe have a physical cause, yet testing fails to produce any evidence of objective biomarkers of a biological abnormality – an illness. It can also be that a treatment appears to work … but that can be sheer chance or the almighty placebo effect.

Some patients, inappropriately assigned a diagnosis in Room 3, may have a diagnosable rare condition that is actually in Room 2, Occult Identifiable Causes. Then again, the underlying cause may simply be undefinable given our current state of knowledge. The mental illness label 'Depression' is one example of a condition that can fit in this category because patients with this "diagnosis"[51] [52] rarely present with concrete evidence of abnormalities of brain chemistry or any other biomarker. It is 'diagnosis by description'.

Despite this, some clinicians speculate, in the absence of evidence, the existence of a cryptic biological abnormality they term "biochemical imbalance"[53]. These patients might or might not have such a problem, but independent evidence supporting the conclusion is absent. Treatment is a shot in the dark! What's worse, many treatments for depression can leave the patient dependent on drugs. The patient must continue medicating forever and sometimes needs to take more and more or yet another medication to address that one's side effects! Withdrawal can be devastating and induce suicidal ideation. The patients are trapped in a vicious circle.

Remember that, when a known biochemical abnormality has been found, the clinician will state exactly which structure, chemical, or hormone is abnormal. Diabetes, thyroid and adrenal diseases all express biochemical abnormalities and patients are normally told the definitive evidence of the problem. If patients are told they have a "biochemical imbalance", they should be told which chemicals are imbalanced and by how much.

LIFESTYLE CHANGE WORKS

In DZ's practice, a patient complained of increasing fatigue and weight gain after her previous doctor had started her on an antidepressant. She related that,

---

51 World Health Organization ICD Classification Bluebook 2018 Codes F32.0 Mild Depressive Episode, F32.1 Moderate Depressive Episode, and F32.3 Severe depressive episode without psychotic symptoms. https://www.icd10data.com/ICD10CM/Codes/F01-F99/F30-F39/F32-/F32.0. Accessed December 7, 2022.

52 DSM V Classification F 32 DSM-5 Update, Supplement to Diagnostic and Statistical Manual of Mental Disorders, Fifth Edition, October 2018, American Psychiatric Association, Washington D.C. https://psychiatryonline.org/pb-assets/dsm/update/DSM5Update_October2018.pdf. Accessed December 7, 2022.

53 It's useful to remember that when doctors identify biochemical abnormalities, for example thyroid, adrenal, or parathyroid imbalances, they state the chemical that is imbalanced and measure chemical or hormone levels to confirm that the treatment is "balancing" the chemical that was imbalanced.

after blood tests, her doctor said she had a "biochemical imbalance" that the antidepressant would correct.

DZ called her previous doctor who reported the patient had complained of feelings of boredom and writer's block. He said that the complete battery of blood work (including hemoglobin, thyroid, and adrenal investigations) was normal. Somehow, he inferred that she had a biochemical imbalance, noting that when she had tried to stop the antidepressant, she felt worse. After considering the lack of evidence for a biochemical disturbance, the patient decided to stop the antidepressant. She did so gradually, over 2 months, substituting a diet and exercise routine. Soon she felt fine and became energetic, and productive, and she has maintained this for the last several years. Note: if she had dropped off the medication precipitously, she would probably have experienced withdrawal symptoms and possibly concluded the antidepressant really was correcting something!

The appropriate treatment of problems like this is symptomatic, that is, the doctor should take steps to ameliorate the symptoms, perhaps based on experience with other similar patients. The physician should start with the least invasive interventions, including psychotherapy, diet and exercise and behavioral therapies. If these less-invasive therapies are not effective, it becomes appropriate to try medical treatments including placebos[54] and, ultimately, psychoactive drugs. An exception might be to intervene pharmaceutically, acutely and temporarily, if the depression is severe and especially if the patient is suicidal, self-destructive or threatening others. Always the warning though: the treatment itself can have side effects that cause other problems or potentiate the chances of suicide!

If our cart is still empty, go out the door on the far wall and into **Room 4 – The Room of Situational Causes**. There is a plethora of possible causes on the shelves here – and the room is vast, as it contains all the myriad ways life disturbs people and relative to which they need support. All we can learn from this room is to treat the patient psychosocially, as it is very likely there is no biological disease, only disappointment, discomfort and dysfunction – all those normal human responses. Peoples' mental states may and often do reflect the normal reaction of the mind and body to life's circumstances.

There are countless Situational Causes. For instance, some children grow up in environments where their caregivers reinforce inappropriate behaviors or do not provide essential emotional sustenance. Grief and post-traumatic reactions are other situations that are emotionally damaging for everyone.

The problems of patients in this category should usually be addressable with psychotherapy and lifestyle interventions; medical intervention should only be a last resort (or used acutely and briefly in the case of severe problems).

It is wise for us to note that knowledge of pharmaceuticals and interventions keep advancing, so there will be exceptions. It is quite possible that in the future a research group will identify safer, non-addictive compounds that help people deal with problems related to their life experiences. Rigorous examination, including clinical trials, can hopefully ensure that these new substances will be effective while not having significant side effects. Of course, we might even find the equivalent of Soma celebrated in Aldous Huxley's Brave New World and *"a gram will be better than a damn".*[55] But don't bet on it!

REHABILITATING STREET DRUGS?

Consider for example, the use of MDMA (3,4-methylenedioxy-methamphetamine, the active ingredient in the street-drug Ecstasy). It has reportedly shown a degree of usefulness as an adjunct to psychotherapy in treating military combatants' post-traumatic

---

54   Roose SP, Rutherford BR, Wall MM, Thase ME. Practising evidence-based medicine in an era of high placebo response: number needed to treat reconsidered. Br J Psychiatry. 2016;208(5):416-420. https://pubmed.ncbi.nlm.nih.gov/27143006/. Accessed December 7, 2022.

55   https://en.wikipedia.org/wiki/Brave_New_World. Accessed December 7, 2022.

stress. "MDMA was first used in the 1970s as an aid in psychotherapy. The drug did not have the support of clinical trials (studies using humans) or approval from the U.S. Food and Drug Administration. In 1985, The U.S. Drug Enforcement Administration labeled MDMA as an illegal drug with no recognized medicinal use. Some researchers remain interested in its value in psychotherapy when given to patients under carefully controlled conditions. MDMA is currently in clinical trials as a possible treatment aid for post-traumatic stress and anxiety in terminally ill patients, and for social anxiety in autistic adults."[56]

Examples of the effects of our experiences, past and present, fill Room 4. Clinicians misdiagnose people as having medical disorders based on what is in this room! The truth is that their mental health problems may just reflect their life experiences. Those who have experienced traumatic events in the past may develop fears that are not appropriate in current circumstances. Sometimes clinicians can even identify the environmental experience that caused the mental health problems and deal with this. Often, people with lifestyle-induced mental health issues are mislabelled with diagnoses from room 3. Later we discuss how we can help each other when lifestyle issues affect us.

On leaving Room 4, if our shopping cart is still empty, we must take the exit door on the far wall. It opens to the Great Outdoors of Mislabelled Causes.

The **Exit to The Great Outdoors of Mislabelled Causes** gives us access to labels (not diagnoses) that characterize people as mentally ill, but where their behaviors are merely out of the comfort zone of some doctors and community members. They are just different. We perceive these people as abnormal or weird, but they may be exhibiting behaviors or thinking that enable them to cope with their own realities and be able to contribute to society in ways that are meaningful

to themselves. Many great scientists, artists and thinkers fit in this category. Consider Dr. Paul A. M. Dirac, the famous Nobel Laureate quantum physicist, whom one biographer classified as exhibiting Asperger's Syndrome, now included in the psychiatric term 'Autism Spectrum Disorder'.[57] If some clinician had curtailed his and others' creativity with drugs, we might have been denied many innovations and much beauty! This should remind clinicians of the dangers of over-diagnosis and warn us regarding the hazards of rushed or biased judgements.

Having arrived here with an empty cart, we can leave the cart behind in the parking lot and accept reality – the patient is just different and neither we nor anyone else should stand in the way!

A BETTER METAPHOR FOR BOOKWORMS

Some readers might prefer the metaphor of a library or a bookstore. Let's instead of our Emporium, imagine a giant bookstore with topics (like bookstores do with Science, English Literature, History and so on) in separate rooms.

In this bookstore we would proceed in the same way as in the Emporium. Room 1 might contain books with information about problems with Identifiable Physiological/Biological Causes. Room 2 would have books addressing problems with Rare Identifiable Causes. Room 3, The Room of Speculative and Unidentifiable Causes, would include books expressing hypotheses, medical fantasies, unfounded claims and many empty shelves waiting for researchers to identify and write about the not yet discovered biological problems that cause mental health disturbances. Room 4, The Room of Situational Causes, would hold books describing how our environment and life context produce mental health problems. The back door of the bookstore might put us in The Great Outdoors to search uselessly and unproductively for information on problems with Mislabeled Causes, when people are given mental health labels but are

---

56 https://www.drugabuse.gov/publications/drugfacts/mdma-ecstasymolly. Accessed December 7, 2022.
57 The Strangest Man, G. Farmelo, Basic Books, Faber and Faber, 2009 ISBN: 978-0-571-22278-0.

happily living productive lives, contributing to the world around them.

We would go into the store, grab a cart, and proceed from room to room in search of books about a specific problem. The problem might be feeling depressed, being unable to sleep or being confused. Books about the problem might be in any or all of the rooms, as something like 'feeling depressed' might have any of those causes.

The additional value of this metaphor is that it emphasizes that what we seek is information, and a bookstore (or library) is a storehouse of information.

Summary

We proffer that the correct causal basis for the mental health problems of all patients is in one of these virtual locations. Clinicians should make an intellectual effort to consider if their patient with mental health issues has: (1) a common, demonstrable medical condition, like thyroid disease; (2) a rare, identifiable, but elusive medical condition the clinician has not yet diagnosed, but that has detectable biomarkers, for example, Addison's Disease; (3) an unidentified but mislabelled hypothetical 'diagnosis' or one that, as yet, is a medically-undiscovered biological condition for which biomarkers might eventually be identified, like an intestinal microbiome-related problem;[58] (4) just normal reactions to his or her life context; or (5) no treatable or treatment-worthy problem and is simply different. In the latter case, it may be that those around the patient are the ones who need help.

58 Deans E. Microbiome and mental health in the modern environment. J Physiol Anthropol. 2016 Jun 27;36(1):1. doi: 10.1186/s40101-016-0101-y. PMID: 27405349; PMCID: PMC4940716. https://www.ncbi.nlm.nih.gov/pmc/articles/PMC4940716/. Accessed December 7, 2022.

Chapter 6: —————— Mental Health Treatment

KEYWORDS: Interventions, Treatment, Placebo, Lifestyle Changes, Verbal Therapy, Behavior Modification, Electroshock Treatment, Surgery

ABSTRACT: We discuss the categories and types of treatment for mental health problems and how treatments, especially initial interventions, should reflect an understanding or lack thereof of the cause. For people with mental symptoms associated with a medical condition, the treatment should be the treatment of that medical condition, augmented by the mental health support needed during recovery. For people where interveners believe a dysfunctional life context is its origin, treatments often involve psychotherapy or various forms of behavioral therapy. For those where the cause is unknown, we endorse initial nonbiological interventions, including talking with people who can help, lifestyle changes, diet and exercise and self- or other-administered rewards and punishments. For people who are unusual but happy with themselves and appreciated by those around them, we advocate avoiding labels and not imposing mental health interventions.

A CLIENT WITH A BAG OF BUGS

A veterinarian had a client who arrived periodically at the clinic complaining of her pet's having infestations of "bugs". In one instance, the client supported this claim by bringing along a shopping bag full of pieces of tape with 'bugs' stuck to them. The veterinarian dutifully examined a sample of the tapes under the microscope and showed the client that there were hairs, dandruff, dirt – or belly button fluff – no bugs! The client left unconvinced and repeatedly returned. This is clearly an issue of the client's mind, is likely harmless and no amount of evidence has proved or would prove convincing. Many physicians have faced similar circumstances where a patient has an imagined symptom that nothing will cure. There are even stories where surgeons have finally given in to a patient's claim that a gremlin of some sort had embedded itself abdominally. They did surgery and told the patient it was removed. Unfortunately, the patient later sought surgery again, claiming the gremlin had returned. Thinking can be disordered!

Sometimes, though, physicians believe that a patient is imagining a problem; they only provide reassurance and find out years later there was a real problem located in Room 2 of the Mental Health Diagnosis Emporium.

Introduction ——————

How do care providers deal with problems with patients' minds? See FIGURE 2.6.1 There's no equivalent of a 'bone spur' and no 'brain appendix' that's inflamed. What can Medicine do about problems of the mind?

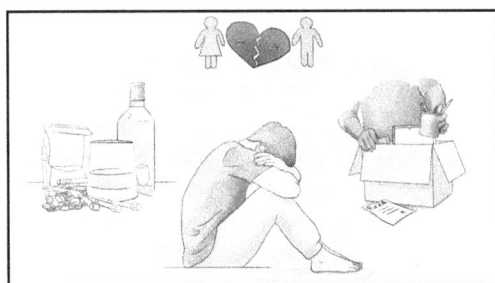

FIGURE 2.6.1: People are Often Surrounded by Social Challenges

Well, there are many ways therapists can help! Luckily, the brain is attached to the ears, eyes and mouth and the mind can access these! In this chapter, we will address a range of mental health therapies and treatments that clinicians and patients can consider when faced with a mental health problem.

Mental Health-related treatment is similar to but a bit different from the usual medical interventions. Some physicians (often Orthopedic Surgeons or Orthopods) set bones and repair injured limbs. Others administer blood and other fluids and apply means of immediate life support (e.g., Emergency Physicians and Intensivists in the ICU). Surgeons perform a variety of internal repairs and other invasive interventions. Virtually all listen, give advice and comfort and prescribe pharmaceuticals.

The care of patients with mental problems, very common visitors to the physician's office, differs in that the penultimate interventions – the listening, advising and comforting – become the crucial ones. Unfortunately, the application of interventions like these is often minimized or sidelined if the physician sees mental problems as only having biological causes (like a damaged or physiologically compromised brain), rather than recognizing that there are problems where thinking is disordered or dysfunctional, despite a perfectly healthy brain. This myopia and tunnel vision can lead to an early flight to drugs.

FOR CLARIFICATION

Please don't get us wrong: Drugs are useful agents in addressing some mental issues but are not always (and maybe never) the complete answer. This is because other side effect-free interventions are often quite effective and essential as adjuncts. Indeed, all of us ordinary people use the same interventions (formally or informally) as those used by mental health experts when we try to influence the thoughts, feelings and behavior of those around us. We listen. We ask lots of gentle questions. We empathize and sympathize.

How Ordinary Humans Behave in Such Circumstances —————

We all have ways of dealing with distressed people. We perhaps ask that the person express and clarify feelings. We try to ameliorate fears or confusion, by providing reassurance. We may suggest things that worked for us or someone we know. We suggest different behaviors including better nutrition and increased fitness. We cajole, we reward and, sometimes, we punish (for example by withholding interaction till the person calms down or by giving a child a time-out). We reinforce that we are there, that we are ready to respond when needed and that we want to help. Whether we can explain mental health problems or not, it is important to understand how to help people with them, and to learn which interventions are effective and which do not work. This means that we might have to develop or get access to more formal knowledge and skills if we want to help people trying to deal with more significant mental health disturbances, including encouraging them to see a professional. Counselors do that. We don't have to be anointed as physicians to do this! And we certainly don't need legal access to a prescription pad.

EFFECTS OF DRUGS

In the case of depression, "It is undesirable to expect 100% treatment coverage for depression, given many will remit before access to services is feasible. Data were drawn from consenting waitlist and primary-care samples, which potentially over-represented mild-to-moderate cases of depression. Considering reported rates of spontaneous remission, a short untreated period seems defensible for this subpopulation, where judged appropriate by the clinician. Conclusions may not apply to individuals with more severe depression."

"Long-term studies show that people are more likely to recover social function if drugs are discontinued early. However, in the existing studies full recovery of vocational and social function (about 20% in people who continue to take prescribed drugs and

40% in people who discontinued prescribed drugs) is not satisfactory."[59]

Moreover, reports of drugs' causing loss of brain grey matter, increased mortality and other health risks, mean that it important to use the least amount of medication and to discontinue medication whenever the benefits of stopping outweigh the potential benefits of continuing.

Recently, the company that manufactures a drug for treating schizophrenia and mania (Risperdal) was assessed and is appealing an 8-billion-dollar settlement because the drug stimulated male breast growth (gynecomastia).[60] Other lawsuits proceeded because patients were not warned of significant side effects including gynecomastia, type 2 diabetes, stoke and cardiac events.[61]

(emphasis ours)

It isn't always easy, though. Sometimes the problems are more serious and not addressable using approaches like those. Often, even experienced clinicians are unable to find a definite cause or any clear solution for the patient's mental problems. The previous chapter recognized that some mental health problems relate to diagnosable and treatable abnormal biology, others relate to abnormal biology that clinicians have not yet discovered, while others do **not** indicate abnormal biology.

With the present state of science, there are many mental health problems that we don't understand, especially when they do not, in fact, have a biological cause. Life events can

be harsh (like seeing a loved one perish in an accident) and our reactions to life events can be dramatic, soul-piercing and enigmatic. Even with a completely normal brain, facing searing memories and untangling and coping with feelings can compromise the strongest person and can require time to develop coping mechanisms. However, usually, even when a biological abnormality has been detected, it is still most appropriate to start with – and continue with – non-pharmacological tools in efforts to improve mental health. Pharmaceuticals are powerful swords that cut both ways. Another analogy: a gun. Shooting it without knowing what you're aiming at is an accident in progress.

Causes of Mental Dysfunction ——

Cause[62] is what connects one process to another. It is usual that multiple elements contribute to mental dysfunction. Although researchers diligently search for physical or biological explanations of mental health abnormalities, many remain unexplained. No one has identified genetic features in people who seem otherwise normal that invariably predict mental health problems. There have been what are called 'whole genome' studies to find associations of mental health problems with specific genes, but these have turned up tens or hundreds of apparent gene associations, with little or no consistency or solid correlations. Indeed, demonstrating genetic links, even

---

59 Whiteford HA, Harris MG, McKeon G, Baxter AJ, Pennell C, Barendregt JJ, Wang JL. Estimating remission from untreated major depression: a systematic review and meta-analysis. Psychological Medicine. August 2012. doi: 10.1017/S0033291712001717. https://www.cambridge.org/core/journals/psychological-medicine/article/estimating-remission-from-untreated-major-depression-a-systematic-review-and-metaanalysis/52961032C5AFAB1C3B2C4E06A652B561. Accessed December 7, 2022.

60 https://www.wsj.com/articles/j-j-hit-with-8-billion-jury-award-over-antipsychotic-drug-11570577281.   Wall Street Journal. January, 18 2020. Accessed December 7, 2022.

61 https://www.consumersafety.org/drug-lawsuits/risperdal/. Accessed December 7, 2022.

62 Something is a cause if its presence is either necessary or sufficient for something else to happen. Drinking water is a necessary condition for living, however, water alone is not enough for life. Other conditions must also be present to cause life to be sustained including air, and food. In mental health an impoverished early childhood, for example, is usually either not necessary or sufficient to produce future mental health abnormalities. The ongoing elements of a person's life and multiple conditions together might to necessary to produce ongoing mental health dysfunction.

where they exist, is exceptionally difficult.[63] On the other hand, some of these searches have uncovered the equivalent of what the police call "persons of interest", if not "suspects". Perhaps we could call them 'causes of interest', or 'possible causes of interest' – but science has not yet been able to pin the definitive label 'perpetrator' (the cause) on them. Except in rare instances, for example Down's Syndrome, no one is yet able to state that specific genes or sets thereof are reliable predictors of one's mental condition.

Our 'spider sense' is tickled regarding genetic causes because we see the familial associations with certain mental problems, like autism and schizophrenia. If, for example, one identical twin has a problem like this, then there is a higher probability that the other of the pair will have it as well. Researchers have reason to search for an identifiable genetic correlate, but there are likely multiple needles in many haystacks, and it will take time to find them.

Furthermore, the task of finding causes for mental health problems is hampered by the difficulty clinicians have applying useful diagnostic labels to the problems. In the case of other kinds of problems, physicians can impugn an invading bacterium and apply the diagnostic label 'Black Plague' or 'Typhoid' and then treat that as the target. There is a clear correlation between the patient's symptoms and findings and the known effects of the invader. Then, focused treatment can be applied that has previously worked on that invader. Researchers try to find treatments by examining the influence they have on people who are like each other in terms of signs, symptoms and findings. The major problem in dealing with mental health is that, often, people with the same symptoms and signs do not have similar origins or causes of these problems. As well, people with the same problem may have different other problems and get differently labelled. It is very difficult to treat when the target is unknown, fuzzy or

multiform! To complicate matters further, behaviors acceptable in one society might be regarded as highly dysfunctional in another.

Mental health problems differ from most medical problems in that we often cannot find a biological cause or there is none. This frustrates doctors, as they should and usually do implement treatments aimed at correcting known biologically caused problems.

Treating Medical Problems That Have Mental Health Symptoms —

There are many examples of mental effects caused by biological illness. We have already mentioned several. Consider that, in addition to those, there are a number of genetically determined metabolic abnormalities that are associated with problems of intellect, mood and conduct. One of these, phenylketonuria (PKU), is an inherited (genetic) disorder that results in the decreased metabolism (breakdown) of the amino acid phenylalanine, a component of many proteins in our food. The accumulation of phenylalanine in the body causes brain and other damage. Infants with PKU develop a build-up of phenylalanine – from the vegetables, meat and breast milk they ingest – and consequently suffer from a variety of physical and mental problems. People with PKU may have behavioral problems and intellectual disability. The treatment, a lifelong diet of foods low in phenylalanine, allows children to avoid the consequences of this genetic defect. Newborn screening for PKU has become routine and, in this case, the treatment prevents the mental consequences of the condition.

Other medical conditions, including, to name a few, the brain tumors, thyroid disease and adrenal disease we have repeatedly mentioned, also cause mental problems. However, these conditions often remain hidden while

---

63   Alexander Arguello, P., Addington, A., Borja, S. *et al.* From genetics to biology: advancing mental health research in the Genomics ERA. Mol Psychiatry 24, 1576–1582 (2019). https://www.nature.com/articles/s41380-019-0445-x. Accessed December 7, 2022.

clinicians attempt to alleviate their troublesome signs and symptoms, which is sometimes like a game of whack-a-mole. The eventual treatment of the disease will, hopefully, ameliorate or terminate its associated mental health symptoms, and the physician will follow up with appropriate psychosocial support, as should be the case with any medical conditions.

However, many mental health problems are simply not associated or yet able to be associated with a well-understood disease. This suggests that clinicians and communities consider a wider range of solutions, not only pharmaceuticals.

PSYCHOSURGERY – A BRAIN-ECTOMY

There is a very famous story about the patient H.M. After years of epileptic seizures that drugs did not control, patient H.M. (Henry Molaison) was subject to brain surgery where a part of his brain was removed. This cured his seizures but left him unable to form near-term memories. He could remember things that happened before his surgery. However, soon after meeting someone new, he had absolutely no memory of that person. This is a very interesting story told in an excellent book: "Patient H.M. – A Story of Madness and Family Secrets", by Luke Dietrich (Chatto and Windus, 2016). It reveals the issues and effects associated with psychosurgery.[64]

Non-drug treatment of Mental Health Problems

Medical doctors, including psychiatrists, have the unique authority to prescribe pharmaceuticals for mental health issues (although in some jurisdictions, other professionals including psychologists and nurses can order a limited range of prescription medications). Other than that, everyone, including mental health workers, can use similar strategies to influence others' mental state. At a simple level, we all use verbal exhortations and some forms of rewards and punishment. Interestingly, we can even self-intervene: some mental health problems improve with better diet and fitness, especially after we resolve to change our behavior.

Even some medical conditions associated with known biomarkers improve when people change their lifestyle and diet. Diabetes and many heart problems are good examples. If patients with Type 2 diabetes can lose a substantial amount of weight, sometimes they can decrease or cease insulin injections. Occasionally, doctors may wait to intervene in the case of even well-defined medical diseases, and people may come to feel better on their own.

People with mental health problems absent a known biological cause can consider a large range of possible assistance and interventions. We have pointed out that, with other than severe mental health problems, it is frequently appropriate to consider verbal therapy as the first choice. Avoiding pharmaceutical intervention, if possible, can be important. This is especially true, as some drug treatments have paradoxical effects. For instance, the decrease in libido and activity that antidepressants often cause is like the common effect of depression.

So, what interventions are possible and appropriate?

INTERVENTIONS IN MENTAL HEALTH – MANOUVERS THAT INFLUENCE THOUGHTS, FEELINGS AND BEHAVIOR

- *General – Sympathetic ear, reinforcing therapist affect and body language, watchful waiting, encourage patient to reflect on solve problem.*
- *Lifestyle Changes – Diet, change of physical environment and relationships and exercise.*
- *Verbal Therapies – Rogerian talk therapy, directive counselling, various schools of psychotherapy, cognitive behavior therapy.*
- *Behavior Modification – Reward and punishment, time outs, approach-avoidance, altering contingencies.*

---

64 Patient H.M.: A Story of Memory, Madness, and Family Secrets, Aug 9, 2016, Random House Publishing, ISBN-13:9780679643807.

- *Drugs – Using chemicals or placebos to change thoughts, feelings and behavior for people with both normal and abnormal biology.*
- *Electrical Techniques– ECT, Low Voltage Transcranial direct current brain stimulation.*[65]
- *Psychosurgery – Prefrontal lobotomy, lesion removal surgery.*

Perhaps the first question we need to consider is to whom we should go to get help if we have a mental problem and we need help. The list below indicates, in no particular order, some of the groups of professionals and just ordinary people who may be able to help. It isn't a short list:

1. Medical Doctors including psychiatrists

2. Psychologists

3. Nurses

4. Social Workers

5. Marriage Counselors

6. Personal Trainers

7. Teachers

8. Social Workers

9. Hypnotherapists

10. Police

11. Clergy

12. Friends

13. Parents

14. Other relatives

That's quite the list and there are others we could add. Perhaps one noteworthy addition should be 'Ourselves'. This means that the resource pool is vast, helpers are not on the endangered species list and reaching out is not a stretch. Whom one chooses is based on personal preference and how serious the problem is. If the matter is critical, especially when it affects our relationships, our work and even our desire to live, then a professional should be sought. If not, almost anyone who cares, and you trust, may be able to help.

We have mentioned before how they can help: the normal human interactions with which we all are familiar. Perhaps most important is the powerful action of <u>listening</u>, active listening bearing empathy and concern. Often a conversation can help – listening plus feedback and listening more. Sometimes just being there can be very effective, sitting side-by-side in silence. At other times, constructive advice can at least indicate reaching out and trying to help. And there are many other possibilities that emerge in the moment and demonstrate that moment is one of caring. These are not highly structured therapeutic interventions that can only be learned in formal training! They are within all of us…if we actually want to make a difference.

Like all the rest of Medicine, the desire we have is to know what works and what doesn't for each person with each kind of problem. To find out, the effects (outcomes) of various interventions must be measured, compared and assessed.

OTHER THOUGHTS

We considered placing the next section earlier in the text, as it is so crucial. However, for readability, we placed it next. The important point is that treatments of all kinds have a purpose and, if we evaluate the state of the person afterward, we can measure if they work. Perhaps a good example is the use of treatment to calm someone, to make them more tranquil or to quiet agitated thinking or feeling. Peace and tranquility are not necessarily the most important measures of success. Sometimes, upset, agitation or appropriate anger is good and more appropriate. Many of us would be sorry to have only calm thoughts when we hear about some of the bizarre activities in the world including dictators' behaviors and the suppression of rights. We really must define the objectives of

65 Lee JC, Lewis CP, Daskalakis ZJ, Croarkin PE. Transcranial Direct Current Stimulation: Considerations for Research in Adolescent Depression. Front Psychiatry. 2017;8: 91. Published 2017 Jun 7. doi:10.3389/fpsyt.2017.00091. https://www.ncbi.nlm.nih.gov/pmc/articles/PMC5461263/. Accessed December 7, 2022.

treatment as being beneficial to the patient or society or, preferably, both. Then we must evaluate the treatment to determine if we achieved our goals.

Measures of Success for Mental Health Interventions

The objective measures of success of interventions in mental health are improved comfort, coherent and appropriate thoughts, positive behaviors, worthwhile overall function, and the overall feeling of being worthwhile and peaceful.

WHAT IS "APPROPRIATE"?

The issue of how to define appropriate thoughts, feelings and behavior is one reason that mental health workers sometimes disagree about the need for intervention. On the other hand, at the extremes of abnormal thinking, emotions and behavior, mental health workers and the public usually agree.

The aim of mental health treatment is to improve mental health and not, as we have stated, changing a biomarker, as there are few, if any, of these. Unfortunately, there are no laboratory tests for 'serum comfort', for example, to see if it has improved. Neither will medical imaging or electroencephalographic (EEG signal) recording or any other test indicate if a person has or has not overcome a mental health problem. The results of treatment, given our current state of knowledge, are subjective for both the patient and the therapist. So, the measure of success is improvement in subjective and objective mental state, not changes in biomarkers.

Contrary to popular belief, clinicians do not measure brain chemicals as part of day-to-day practice and are not able to find out if treatments corrected aberrant brain chemistry. However, we must always recognize that people may have undetected (but possibly detectable) or unknown biochemical abnormalities. Instead, clinicians measure the effectiveness of interventions, including if drugs have improved things, by using self-report, observation, enquiry and other information provided by the patient, friends, employers and relatives to evaluate changes. Successful treatments are ones where the patient and those around the person agree there has been an improvement. Of course, if they want to, people can report and act that they are now fine, sometimes just to escape the treatment process itself!

Treatments in Mental Health

Most people are familiar with the use of medication to treat known illnesses. They are less familiar with the use of psychoactive agents as a therapeutic trial to help a problem that has proved refractory to psychotherapy and other non-pharmaceutical maneuvers, even when the cause of the problem is not known.

Therapeutic Trial of a Psychoactive Agent

Clinicians recognize that there are many types of intervention available for mental health problems, including pharmaceuticals. When non-pharmacological interventions fail, it is sometimes worthwhile to consider a 'therapeutic trial' of a drug. This is used when the physician believes but has not confirmed that a patient has a specific condition. For example, a doctor might consider prescribing an antidepressant. In a therapeutic trial, the doctor will prescribe the antidepressant to see if it helps, even in the short-term. If the patient improves, the therapeutic trial was successful, although there is no way to know for sure if the antidepressant was what really made a difference. In a sense, it may not matter, considering the patient feels better. One issue here, though, is that antidepressants and other psychoactives may take a while to have an effect and they can cause unpleasant side effects that can make the situation worse. Further, the effects of withdrawal from the agent after the trial can be nasty and other drugs may be piled on to deal with that.

The problem with this approach is that the situation can easily spiral out of control.

'Watchful Waiting' is another form of therapeutic trial. The assumption is that the problem is self-limited, that the feeling or dysfunction will pass. In the case of mental health problems, a clinician might try a safe intervention – for example prescribing diet, exercise and counselling – to see if the person improves on his or her own with that bit of help. If there is improvement with non-medicinal interventions, the patient will have avoided the possible adverse reactions or bad side effects of medication. They also do not have withdrawal symptoms. That's why this is a good way to start.

IMPORTANT NOTE

The treatments discussed in this chapter are for mental problems. The chapter assumes that the clinician has ordered and reviewed the results of appropriate tests for medical conditions that have associated mental health problems and that these results show no objective evidence of abnormal body chemistry or of brain abnormalities.

Furthermore, they assume that the patient is not an immediate threat to self or others. In that emergent situation, safety is likely the primary concern and time is not wasted in addressing matters effectively.

Why Watchful Waiting and Therapeutic Trials Can be Good Ideas

To make it clear why watchful waiting is wise, it is worthwhile realizing that over 50% of people with major depression recover within a year without treatment.[66] Also, over 70% of people with mental health problems reasonably successfully seek informal help, usually from friends, family and religious leaders.[67] Fewer than 30% seek expert advice, although people with more complicated and severe problems do appropriately tend to consult professionals.

Unfortunately, we do not know if patients who start with informal advice have better long-term results compared with those who immediately seek more formal care. Researchers have not done the studies to find that out. The high spontaneous recovery rate from mental health problems does at least suggest that watchful waiting is often a highly appropriate strategy for mild to moderate mental struggles. Sometimes, though, the struggle is more concerning, as in the case of the threat of suicide or homicide.

Suicide is a serious problem and is increasingly common in many jurisdictions. However, no well-designed research has answered the very important question: Does psychiatric intervention reduce or increase the chances of suicide? This is not surprising because patients are so varied, as are the beliefs of their care providers. There has been recent work monitoring people's moods using electronic device-supported apps and there is a degree of success claimed (but not cogently substantiated) by the app developers in predicting suicidal crises. However, only scientific trials will show the true value of approaches like this. Studies of the use of devices are frustrated by many factors, including patients' negative reactions to technology, the dispiriting nature of mental problems that deter commitment to the discipline required, worry that confidentiality might be compromised, fears that suicidal risk will be increased by focusing an individual on the problem and even by Luddism. Electronic

---

66   Whiteford HA, Harris MG, McKeon G, Baxter A, Pennell C, Barendregt JJ, Wang J., Estimating remission from untreated major depression: a systematic review and meta-analysis, Psychol Med. 2013 Aug;43(8):1569-85. doi: 10.1017/S0033291712001717. Epub 2012 Aug 10. https://www.ncbi.nlm.nih.gov/pubmed/22883473. Accessed December 7, 2022.

67   Brown, J.S., Evans-Lacko, S., Aschan, L, et. Al. Seeking informal and formal help for mental health problems in the community: a secondary analysis from a psychiatric morbidity survey in South London, BMC Psychiatry 2014, 14:275. https://pubmed.ncbi.nlm.nih.gov/25292287/ . Accessed December 7, 2022.

devices are perceived by many as invasive. We will have to see how these efforts progress.

IMPORTANT REFERENCES

Nature vol 563 Nov 2018 pp 20 – 22

https://www.scientificamerican.com/article/suicide-risk-assessment-doesnt-work/. Accessed December 7, 2022.

https://www.nature.com/articles/s41380-019-0531-0 Accessed December 7, 2022.

Nature Suicide Prediction Models Don't work.

DR. THOMAS INSEL'S FRAMEWORK

Towards the end of writing this book, Dr. Tom Insel, the former Director of the U. S. National Institute of Mental Health, published the book "Healing: Our Path from Mental Illness to Mental Health" (Penguin Press, 2022). Though still using the term mental 'illness', Dr. Insel offered a very valuable framework for recovery from mental health problems. He called those "The 3 Ps" (esp. pgs. 160-175), standing for People, Place and Purpose. People are friends and community we require for quality living. Place is where we can live and belong. And Purpose is having a reason to recover and live. This is an excellent book and well worth reading.

When Intervention is Important —

We must be aware, however, that people whose behavior is bizarre, threatening or dangerous are in another category. This is because mental health workers and police must consider the safety of the community, as well as the life of the person whose behavior is unacceptable and possibly dangerous. What's more, what may amount to eccentric behaviors can expose a vulnerable mentally unstable person to a life-threatening situation. This is a horrible reality! It happens often that execution (sometimes termed 'suicide by cop') is the penalty for deviant behaviors! The fact is that, sometimes, police feel compelled to use lethal force to protect the public or themselves from people they perceive as threatening. For folks like this, incarceration in a mental institution or a jail or the use of appropriate drugs, not mortal intervention, can help and should happen. However, sometimes one of these non-lethal options is not available or possible. More about this later (See the chapter on Dangerousness).

Discovering How Drugs Work —

Researchers and pharmaceutical companies try to understand how drugs work and they often speculate on mechanisms of action. Usually, in mental health, the speculations relate to changes in brain neurotransmitters (biochemicals that act at the neurons' synapses), including serotonin. However, tests that would support these speculations are not yet available before or after treatment for individuals with mental health problems. We must reemphasize that we are not yet able to determine if a person has a biochemical problem that is causing a mental health aberration or that treatment corrected it, even when pharmaceuticals seem effective. Remember: When a headache resolves with the use of acetaminophen, it does not mean the person had an acetaminophen deficiency.

HAVE PHARMACEUTICALS HIJACKED MENTAL HEALTH CARE?

The problem is that, in dealing with even the more common and less serious mental health problems, psychoactive medications are often the 'go to' intervention. This has stimulated many academics and mental health practitioners to recognize and persistently object to the overuse of psychoactive drugs. Offhandedly prescribing these medications puts people at risk of unnecessary and undesirable complications, including addiction and drug withdrawal problems. For knowledgeable and concerned practitioners, this is a frustration; unfortunately, is also a day-to-day reality.

Formally Evaluating Mental Health Treatments: A Statistical Process

The lack of objective biomarkers of the causes of mental health problems precludes patients or clinicians from objectively measuring either the patient's initial physiological state or determining if an intervention has caused any subsequent physiological change. Therefore, evaluating mental health interventions for individuals requires measuring changes in the patient's feelings, thinking and behaviors. Overall, assessing the effects of treatment is a statistical-association challenge, not a direct cause-and-effect determination. This is a clarion call to health informaticians, researchers, clinicians and administrators. We must develop and use formal, validated, subjective and objective measurement 'instruments' of mental health to learn if an intervention or set of interventions is helpful or harmful. These instruments would use questioning or psychosocial observation and assessment techniques tested by researchers to ensure that they yield meaningful, repeatable and reliable results when applied to different patients in different settings.

Summary

We hope it is clear by now that pharmaceuticals or other invasive interventions are not the only – nor should they be the first – approach to helping most patients with mental health problems. These agents change the mental state of everybody, but they should ideally be used when there is a biological problem that they are designed to correct or when other, less risky, measures have failed. Regretfully, some clinicians go there despite insufficient evidence of effectiveness, and they ignore other methods that could work as well or better.

Any intervenor, especially but not limited to qualified clinicians, can often influence problem behaviors through discussion, persuasion, comforting presence and by using personal rewards (such as praise) and punishments (such as admonishment). Occasionally, however, the safest techniques to change behavior do not work and medicinal interventions become worthy of a trial. Medications, however, should not be a short cut or a quick fix that postpones or substitutes for human-human therapeutic engagement.

Another factor is the variability of patients' responses to drugs, as they are not precise interventions. Consider that some children labelled with the psychiatric diagnosis ADHD (Attention Deficit/Hyperactivity Disorder), when treated with stimulants, appear to improve in their school functioning but not all do. However, stimulants also seem to improve learning and retention in people without ADHD. This might be a problem! Adolescents and others are using neuro-enhancers to improve school and other performance. Amphetamines, intended as a treatment but harboring many potential negative effects, have effectively become street drugs. Physicians, hoping to advantage their patients, often require little provocation to use their prescription pads to improve school performance. They have become dealers!

A POSITIVE EFFECT OF REMOVING CONTROLS?

A pharmacist told DZ that one of the benefits for pharmacists of less rigorous control of amphetamines is that "speed freaks" (her words) no longer harass pharmacists for drugs, nor do they attempt to break into pharmacies to get amphetamines. Rather, they can describe a set of symptoms to doctors and receive legitimate prescriptions.

Chapter 7: ————— The Nature of Psychoactive Drugs

KEYWORDS: Drugs, Psychosis, Decreased Drive, Decreased Behavior, Manifestations of Mental Health Problems

ABSTRACT: Drugs influence mental and physical health in people who have normal or abnormal biology. Many psychoactive drugs can affect abnormal behavior but might reduce normal activities as well. The label 'Attention Deficit/ Hyperactivity Disorder' may help clarify some of the issues. Its frequently pre-scribed treatment, Ritalin, an amphetamine-like drug, seems to increase a person's activity and concentration. Because of its effect on concentration and on engage-ment in learning, students, likely without any biological or mental health abnor-mality, sometimes request the drug to improve their school performance. We must be aware, though, that most drugs, including those prescribed for mental health problems, produce adverse effects. Examples of these untoward effects include involuntary tremors, fatigue, changes in libido and changes in appetite with associ-ated weight gain or loss.

Introduction ————————————

In centuries past, people perceived as having mental symptoms fared badly. Often, they were locked up, sometimes for their whole lives. While they were incarcerated, their keepers subjected them to awful 'treatments'. They were wrapped in blankets and doused with ice-water, bound and gagged, sometimes they had holes drilled into their skulls (trepanation) to 'allow evil to escape' and they were also pun-ished. It took many centuries until they were treated more humanely as disturbed human beings. Unfortunately, questionable measures, like psychosurgery – removal of parts of the brain – were still used even into the last century and psychoactive drugs continue to be over-prescribed.[68]

Today, people with mental health problems are treated far better. At least it seems that way! This is not the case for those unfortunates who are incarcerated in prisons because of crimes, or who end up living on the street without any help whatever. Some people are incarcerated in mental hospitals for treatment after having been declared not-criminally-responsible, even when there have been few efforts to assess the evidence that provoked the initial criminal charge. Reality is that many innocents have found themselves incarcerated after they were stigmatized with a mental health label.[69] Then

68 Bobo WV, Grossardt BR, Lapid MI, et al. Frequency and predictors of the potential overprescribing of antidepressants in elderly residents of a geographically defined U.S. population. Pharmacol Res Perspect. 2019;7(1): e00461. Published 2019 Jan 23. doi:10.1002/prp2.461. https://pubmed.ncbi.nlm.nih.gov/30693088/. Accessed December 7, 2022.

69 Wold, N., 10 Crazy Cases of People Wrongfully Committed to Insane Asylums, ListVerse, Health, Last updated July 20, 2109. https://listverse.com/2015/07/24/10-crazy-cases-of-people-wrongfully-committed-to-insane-asylums/. Accessed December 7, 2022.

there are those prescribed powerful drugs to suppress undesirable symptoms but that reduce them to virtual zombies.

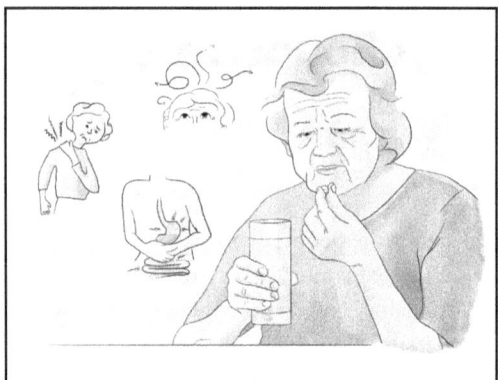

FIGURE 2.7.1: Medicines Often Affect Both the Body and the Mind

Psychiatric Drugs May Reduce Overall Activity, Both Harmful and Useful.

At the minimum, many psychotropic pharmaceuticals tend to reduce activity, interaction and the ability to truly enjoy living. Partly this is due to their origins. Consider that pharmaceutical companies first marketed the psychoactive drug Chlorpromazine (CPZ) as a sedative or an anesthetic before trying it on schizophrenic or psychotic patients – and sedation is often a common side effect of many antipsychotics. Although antipsychotics do reduce abnormal behavior, they also reduce drive. They can make it more difficult for many medicated people to go to school, to work or to have normal interactions with friends and relatives. Sometimes these side effects are significant and themselves engender further treatment. A good example is 'tardive dyskinesia' – random, involuntary movements of parts of one's face or arms and hands often very disturbing to bystanders – a side effect of some psychotropics. FIGURE 2.7.1. illustrates some of the undesired effects of psychotropic drugs.

There are appropriate and acceptable at times for the application of pharmaceuticals to deal with extreme and possibly harmful manifestations of aberrant thinking, anxiety and behavior. However, intervening this way can also have adverse consequences and achieve varying degrees of success – and it is not guaranteed to help. It is incumbent on the prescriber to consider carefully and thoughtfully evaluate the chances of an overall positive effect on behavior versus undesirable effects on the whole patient and bystanders. It is also necessary to follow-up patients carefully to learn about drug effects. It is not appropriate nor enough to consider only the reduction in the patient's undesirable speech, odd behaviors and other unwelcome activities that may disturb others without considering the impact of the intervention on other important aspects of the patient's life.

People labeled 'psychotic' often appear to be out of touch with the environment in which they live. Their behavior may be bizarre. They might report hearing things that are not there and believing things that are not so. Reported hallucinations might be auditory, for example hearing a voice telling them to cross the street or to harm someone. People reporting visual hallucinations might claim to have seen a long-deceased relative or a ghost or phantasm. Someone might also claim to be the Queen of England or Jesus Christ or to have tremendous wealth, even though actually being of modest means. Mental health workers attach the label 'psychosis' to people who have such delusions (beliefs contradicted by generally accepted reality or reason).

Unfortunately, there are no objective tests that will tell the clinician if a person actually experienced a delusion or hallucination or is merely claiming to have heard or seen something. There is simply no way to confirm or deny such a claim unless there is some acting out. Hallucinations are the subjective experience of the patient and are not accessible to external review or evaluation. Clearly, claims of being someone else or of having special powers or abilities can be checked to learn if they are accurate or not (except for politicians who oft get away with such unsubstantiated claims). Of course, interventions are necessary when someone reports that visions are provoking unrealistic fear or impelling the person to take flight from the roof of a building.

Psychiatric Symptoms Sometimes Disturb Communities

Hallucinations or delusions are worrisome to communities and neighbors when they lead to bad behavior. The bad behavior is the real problem, not the hallucinations or delusions. Many of us have fantasies – the authors believe they can write, for example! Normally, we do not mind if someone daydreams, enjoys a pleasant fantasy, paints or writes with the belief that people will like what they do.

If the delusion, hallucination or another severe mental health problem is troubling to the patient or the community, doctors may appropriately suggest interventions, sometimes including pharmaceuticals. They do this when the person or community perceives the problem as serious and when other maneuvers have failed. For serious mental health problems that are resistant to other maneuvers, people should be prepared to accept the unavoidable risks of drug treatments.

Those who take psychotropic medications prescribed by psychiatrists or other clinicians often have the same problems starting or stopping as people have with street drugs. Many psychotropics are addictive because they engender dependence, and withdrawal can be distressing. Further, though their good effects can take time to develop, adverse effects can start immediately. These adverse effects include:

> **Habituation,** where a previously effective drug gradually or quickly loses its effectiveness.

> **Addiction,** where chronic use of a drug creates dependency, often requiring increasing dosage to have the same effects, and it causes withdrawal symptoms on discontinuation.

> **Dependence,** where withdrawal brings back the problem the drug was meant to solve.

> **Motor Retardation,** where energy and activity are reduced.

> **Sexual Dysfunction,** where libido and sexual performance are depressed.

These are not pleasant or even desirable! So, this intervention has risks. However, it is possible a clinician might prescribe a drug for its side effects – perhaps to relax or activate the patient.

TOOLS TO CHANGE FEELINGS

People take either prescription or street drugs to feel differently. We have mentioned that students may show improved intellectual performance[70] – or just perceive that they do – from taking amphetamines, even though they had no biological abnormalities to start with and regardless of the source of the drugs. Some feel amphetamines improve cognitive performance, but if they do, the evidence indicates that it is a minimal improvement.[71] Whatever their actual effectiveness, many students request these drugs from physicians to give them a competitive advantage for university admission or for scholarships. Some ethicists argue that there is little difference between the use of steroids to improve athletic performance and the use of amphetamines to improve academic performance. In both cases, drug users gain a competitive advantage; in both cases, they take risks.

---

70 Wood S, Sage JR, Shuman T, Anagnostaras SG. Psychostimulants and cognition: a continuum of behavioral and cognitive activation. Pharmacol Rev. 2013;66(1):193–221. Published 2013 Dec 16. doi:10.1124/pr.112.007054. https://www.ncbi.nlm.nih.gov/pmc/articles/PMC3880463/. Accessed December 7, 2022.

71 https://www.sciencedirect.com/science/article/abs/pii/S0028390812003577. Accessed December 7, 2022.

A drug that changes thinking, feeling or behaving is not an indicator that there was an underlying biologic abnormality causing a mental problem. Drugs simply change things for good or for bad.

AN EXAMPLE: ATTENTION DEFICIT HYPERACTIVITY DISORDER

Clinicians give children and adults the psychiatric label 'Attention Deficit/Hyperactivity Disorder' (ADHD) when people believe their behavior is not appropriate and perceive it as disruptive. The diagnosis is one of the most common psychiatric labels, even though it is based on "subjective assessments of perceived behavior". [72]

Like many other labels that mental health clinicians use, this is a subjective one that reflects the belief that someone should be more focused on a specific activity. Different people, expert or not, often have different interpretations of the same behavior. Some describe certain behaviors in children as explorations and evidence of curiosity; others consider the same behavior as evidence of a disorder. The diagnosis is often based on the context of the child and on the beliefs of the teachers and the parents. In areas where teachers are more likely to attribute ADHD to younger children in a grade, clinicians are more likely to accept the label as a diagnosis and prescribe drugs. Younger children may only appear to be more active and undisciplined because they are when compared to older, perhaps more mature, children in the grade.

There is poor agreement on how diagnosticians should apply this label. Sometimes physicians distinguish between 'Hyperactive Disorder' and 'Attention Deficit Disorder'. The American Psychiatric Association remarked "[the existence of the two] subtypes of predominantly Hyperactive-Impulsive and predominantly Inattentive ADHD (attention deficit hyperactivity disorder) have [sic] not been supported by the empirical data; instead, the evidence suggests that the classification of subtypes in

ADHD is strongly influenced by method variance (e.g., by differences in informants, instruments, or in the algorithms used for combining information across informants). The consensus is that the existing sub typology is not useful." [73]

The simple translation of the psychiatric jargon above is that the separate terms may not be useful diagnostically or for determining treatment. It indicates that the label used may reflect who uses the terms or the testing instrument. Indeed, teachers and other school personnel, not physicians, are usually the first to suggest the diagnosis of ADHD. [74]

Attention Deficit Hyperactivity Disorder, like many other psychiatric descriptors, is not a diagnosis that usually relies on objective assessment or measurement of behavior. Rather, the label often reflects what people subjectively perceive, expect or tolerate. This places ADHD, unless severe, in the 'Great Outdoors' in the previous chapter.

Modifying Behavior in ADHD ——

Unfortunately, using psychiatric labels as a shortcut to describe people who behave badly may interfere with efforts to implement worthwhile interventions.

Rather than just labelling, it would be better to describe the behavior and the circumstances associated with bothersome behaviors. Is it the home? Is it too much isolation and interacting only with video games? Is it the school? Is it the neighborhood? Is it the effect of unsavory friends? Defining the context, form and possible other environmental causes of perceived misbehavior often leads to non-pharmaceutical interventions and a clear definition of what the interventions are meant to accomplish. Credible research supports that *"ADHD behavioral therapy may be more effective than drugs*

---

72 Gualtieri CT, Johnson LG. ADHD: Is Objective Diagnosis Possible? Psychiatry (Edgmont). 2005;2(11):44-53. https://www.ncbi.nlm.nih.gov/pmc/articles/PMC2993524/. Accessed December 7, 2022.

73 http://www.dsm5.org/progressreports/pages/0904dsm-vadhdanddisruptivebehaviordisordersworkgroup.aspx. Accessed December 7, 2022.
    American Psychiatric Association, DSM 5 Development April 2009, F.X. Casterllanos, accessed July 14, 2015.

74 L. Sax and K. J. Kautz, Who First Suggests the Diagnosis of Attention-Deficit/Hyperactivity Disorder Ann Fam Med. 2003 Sep; 1(3): http://www.ncbi.nlm.nih.gov/pmc/articles/PMC1466583/. Accessed December 7, 2022.

in the long run".[75] The success of behavioral therapies depends on the ability of people to influence other people through rewards and disincentives. Can a teacher ignore inappropriate behavior until the student stops and then reward the calm after the storm? Are children who view the behavior of overactive children encouraging their behavior by laughing, smiling or otherwise approving?

The Centers for Disease Control and Prevention (CDC) suggests that behavioral therapy should be the intervention of first choice, and it describes programs and effective interventions to improve behavior and concentration[76]. Behavioral therapists recognize that certain situations promote abnormal behavior in the home and elsewhere. The CDC recommends well-accepted and recognized maneuvers that are effective and help reduce inappropriate or disruptive behavior and improve concentration.[77] It also recommends that parents learn the skills required to help their children think and behave in better ways. This should be part of the curriculum in parenting, if only there were one.

Unfortunately, the bluntest approach is to make certain behaviors illegal and to link the behaviors with punishments like a fine or jail.

This can reduce those behaviors. Adolescents are less likely to drink excessively in communities where underage and high-volume drinking is illegal.[78] Proceeding less invasively, like having a timeout or removing children briefly from a circumstance in which their behavior is persistently disruptive, can also be effective.

The Harvard Business Review[79] reports several simple maneuvers to change behavior. One way is to change the environment. If it takes more effort to do something, the activity is less likely – adolescents are also less likely to drink if they live further from a liquor store.[80] Moving food away from the immediate environment reduces eating. Consider also that people eat more soup when it is served in a larger bowl and they eat less from smaller bowls.

The Centre for Research in Family Health at Dalhousie University, led by psychologist Dr. Pat McGrath[81], is building on early work[82] demonstrating that simple and timely guidance enables parents to have a major influence on the behavior of children labeled with Attention Deficit or Hyperactivity Disorder. The Centre encourages parents to call at the time the child is misbehaving, and a therapist makes real-time suggestions on how to influence the behavior.

75 SciCurious, Not-So-Quick Fix: ADHD behavioral therapy may be more effective than drugs in the long run, scientific American, May 15, 2012. http://www.scientificamerican.com/article/adhd-behavioral-therapy-more-effective-drugs-long-term/. Accessed December 7, 2022.

76 Attention-Deficit/Hyperactivity Disorder, Centres for Disease Control and Prevention, http://www.cdc.gov/ncbddd/adhd/treatment.html. Accessed November 8, 2016.

77 Attention-Deficit/Hyperactivity Disorder, Centres for Disease Control and Prevention, http://www.cdc.gov/ncbddd/adhd/treatment.html. Accessed November 8, 2016.

78 Journal of American College Health, Vol. 50, No. 5, March 2002 Underage College Students' Drinking Behavior, Access to Alcohol, and the Influence of Deterrence Policies Findings From the Harvard School of Public Health College Alcohol Study, Henry Wechsler; Jae Eun Lee; Toben F. Nelson; Meichun Kuo. https://www.tandfonline.com/doi/abs/10.1080/07448480209595714 . Accessed December 7, 2022.

79 Bregman, P., the easiest way to change people's behavior, Harvard Business Review, March 12, 2009. https://hbr.org/2009/03/the-easiest-way-to. Accessed December 7, 2022.

80 Bregman, P., the easiest way to change people's behavior, Harvard Business Review, March 12, 2009. https://hbr.org/2009/03/the-easiest-way-to. Accessed December 7, 2022.

81 Centre for Research in Family Health. http://crfh.ca/. Accessed July 16, 2016.

82 Pisterman, S., McGrath, P., Fireston, P., et. Al., Outcome of Parent-mediated treatment of preschoolers with attention deficit disorder with hyperactivity, Journal of consulting and clinical psychology 1989, Vol. 57, 5, 628-635. https://www.researchgate.net/profile/Patrick_McGrath/publication/20362428_Outcome_of_parent-mediated_treatment_of_preschoolers_with_attention_deficit_disorder_with_hyperactivity/links/00b4951c60ffed0641000000.pdf. Accessed December 7, 2022.

Their work demonstrates that it is important to establish a clear and immediate link between behavior and consequences, to provide rewards for good behavior and to administer punishment (including time-outs) for poor behavior. For children labeled as hyperactive, the measures of the success of the intervention include an increase in worthwhile behavior, a decrease in disruptive behavior and an increase in compliance with appropriate parent and teacher requests. Successful models for behavioral change recognize that behavior does not occur in a vacuum. The fact is that teacher and parent behavior influence the child, and the child's behavior also has a reflexive important influence on the parent or teacher. Child and authority behaviors are not independent, and interventions must address them together.

Strategies to change the behavior of those around us are part of our lives. These strategies work for children as well. Changing behavior, however, requires very clear objectives and clear instructions.

Consider that many parents see and react to a room full of toys scattered about as a sign of the child's inattention. However, giving the child suggestions to improve neatness are more likely to succeed than the typical: "Clean up the mess!" This is less specific and less successful than "put your dolls in the toy box" might be (although, as parents, it is also valuable to recognize that kids increase entropy – disorder – by nature!). How people communicate with each other does have a major influence on the effectiveness of requests and on subsequent behavior. However, immediate consequences are more effective than delayed ones in influencing behavior. It is counterintuitive but also useful to recognize that intermittent rewards seem to be most effective at maintaining desired behavior.[83] It is not necessary to reward every desired behavior. In fact, it can reduce

the effectiveness of the maneuver. This also works with pets!

There are many kinds of rewards. They include material rewards, such as toys or money, and personal rewards, including attention or praise from a parent or a superior. They might also include access to rewarding activities, for example, time with video games or television, being allowed to attend a performance of the Muppets or just showing interest. Both adults and children value attention from the people around them. An adult who pays attention and is effusive when a child does something worthwhile, makes it more likely that the child will repeat the useful behavior. We see this in dealing with pets. It isn't effective to chide Poopsie after finding a mess. But a treat is a powerful stimulant for getting her to roll over. Just paying attention to the pet garners a positive response. Children (and even peers) can gain from the same considerations we give to simple animals!

Simple and consistent rules are crucial when dealing with aberrant behavior in children or adults. A timeout is a worthwhile distractor and an acceptable punishment for most bad behavior. During a timeout, parents ask a child to go to a different room or they ignore the child for a short period. Timeouts are also effective for adults, which is one reason that companies occasionally suspend workers, with or without pay, for poor performance or misdemeanors. Just suggesting that an aggressive co-worker take a few minutes to think or to come back later is similar. In the case of societally unacceptable behavior, incarceration is another form of timeout.

Why spend so much time on this? Well, it shows that many strategies work to change behavior. What is clear is that in many cases, behavioral therapy, involving talking or using rewards and punishments, is often more effective than using pharmaceuticals to treat people

---

83   http://www.psywww.com/intropsych/ch05-conditioning/index.html. Accessed December 7, 2022.

described as having ADHD or impulsive behavior.[84] The Centers for Disease Control notes there is *"too little behavior therapy for kids with ADHD"*[85] [86]

Although there are many people who speculate that ADHD reflects a medical or biochemical disorder, the fact that lots of people improve with non-medicinal treatment suggests that aberrant biochemistry is not their dominant problem. More usually, the abnormal behavior mirrors an environment that supports rather than discourages unfocused or erratic behavior. It is an important conclusion that people labelled with ADHD respond to the same rewarding and punishing maneuvers as people who do not have the label.

Antipsychotic Drug Treatment ——

Ideas divorced from reality are only truly bothersome when they interfere with a person's ability to care for themselves, prevent them from functioning in the ways they wish, negatively affect the people around them or lead to aggression and violence that can harm themselves or others.

Interventions aimed at reducing psychotic thinking are measured by a reduction in bothersome behaviors, including decreases in the person's claims to hallucinating or other aberrant thinking.

We need to remember that there can be biological causes of aberrant thinking. Oft-mentioned brain tumors, abnormal brain development and metabolic illnesses may cause disordered thinking and behavior. Sometimes, the brain abnormalities result from the abuse of recreational or even prescribed drugs. If that is the case, removing or halting the insult often leads to improved behavior and thinking. Frequently, however, the aberrant thinking does not have a biological cause and can be a reaction to the person's circumstances or experiences. It also may be impossible to assess or measure aberrant thinking. Aberrant behavior, on the other hand, is easily observable.

The evidence is suggestive but not conclusive that, in the last 60 years, as pharmaceuticals became increasingly available, the proportion of people diagnosed as psychotic increased.[87] How much the availability of drugs contributed here is not known, but there seems to be a correlation. In this era, it is easy to recommend drugs to change a patient's mental state. Physicians who concluded that disordered behavior and thinking are 'illnesses' also became more likely to recommend medications as a solution. One psychiatrist remarked that the only major advance in Psychiatry in the last 50 years was the availability of psychotropics and that their prescription now was 50% of psychiatric treatment.[88]

Regrettably, clinicians normally do not track people who are non-compliant with prescribed recommendations. Consequently, we cannot identify the group of non-compliers whose outcomes were better or worse than expected. It is also difficult for researchers

84 Not-So-Quick Fix: ADHD Behavioral Therapy May Be More Effective Than Drugs in Long Run. Cognitive and behavioral therapies that help young people reduce impulsivity and cultivate good study habits are costlier and take longer to administer but may be more efficacious over time. By SciCurious May 15, 2012. https://www.scientificamerican.com/article/adhd-behavioral-therapy-more-effective-drugs-long-term/. Accessed December 7, 2022.

85 CDC Centers for Disease Control and Prevention, Attention-Deficit/Hyperactivity Disorder. Accessed November 9 2016. http://www.cdc.gov/ncbddd/adhd/treatment.html. Accessed December 7, 2022.

86 Too Little Behavioral Therapy for Kids With ADHD. JAMA. 2015;313(20):2016. doi:10.1001/jama.2015.4969. http://jamanetwork.com/journals/jama/article-abstract/2297179. Accessed December 7, 2022.

87 Kirkbride, J.B., Errazuriz, A.K. Croudace, T.J. et al., systematic review of the incidence and prevalence of schizophrenia and other psychoses in England, January 2012, research conducted for the British Department of health policy research program. http://www.psychiatry.cam.ac.uk/files/2014/05/Final-report-v1.05-Jan-12.pdf. Accessed December 7, 2022.

88 Dominic Covvey Personal Communication with R. Campbell.

to track people to find out what happens to those who were <u>not</u> prescribed mind-altering substances to treat an initial episode of bizarre thinking and behavior. Are people better off with or without drugs? Who is most likely to benefit? Who is most likely to be harmed? We simply do not know, but these are important questions that need answers!

Problem is that Antipsychotics Can be Dangerous

For older people with dementia, antipsychotic medication may be deadly. A USA Veterans Administration study[89] reported that, depending on which antipsychotic medication used, the Number Needed to Harm (using death as the measure of harm) varied on average between one out of 26 patients treated to one out of 50. This means that, depending on the antipsychotic used, for every 100 veterans receiving it, between two and four would be more likely to die in the first 180 days of drug treatment. Moreover, people on antipsychotic medication were more likely to die compared with those who took other psychiatric drugs that also reduce activity.[90] [91]

A Danish study concluded *"Antipsychotic drugs on the Danish market today* [2009] *have a very low therapeutic value and seem to be primarily harmful to the patients. From an ethical perspective, antipsychotic drugs can therefore **not** be used as a standard treatment for any mental illness. Further scientific investigation into the significance of this finding is urgently needed. Antipsychotic drugs might still be justified in the treatment of specific subgroups of patients like violent and sexually aggressive, acute psychotic, schizophrenic patients."* [92] (Emphasis and insertion ours).

Proper studies that track the characteristics and fate of people who take antipsychotic medication are essential to learn who is more likely to benefit or be harmed. Long-term studies are essential because effects can be delayed; capturing the detailed (and changing) characteristics of people treated can be challenging too. There is another problem. A Cochrane Collaboration Review[93] that compared antipsychotics recognized that many people prescribed antipsychotics stopped them early. These dropouts make it difficult to complete such long-term studies with adequate numbers. Patients are more likely to stop taking conventional antipsychotics because they are associated with a variety of side effects including weight gain and serious metabolic problems. Moreover, many who stop early are better off.[94]

Tom Insel, the Director of the National Institute of Mental Health (NIMH) in the

89   Maust DT, Kim HM, Seyfried LS, et.al., Antipsychotics, other psychotropics and the risk of death in patients with dementia: number needed to harm. JAMA Psychiatry. 2015 May;72(5):438-45. doi: 10.1001/jamapsychiatry.2014.3018. http://www.ncbi.nlm.nih.gov/pubmed/25786075. Accessed December 7, 2022.

90   A. G. Szmulewicz; F. Angriman; F. E. Pedroso; C. Vazquez; and D. J. Martino, Long-Term Antipsychotic Use and Major Cardiovascular Events: A Retrospective Cohort Study, J Clin Psychiatry 2017;78(8): e905–e912. https://www.psychiatrist.com/jcp/article/Pages/2017/v78n08/16m10976.aspx. Accessed December 7, 2022.

91   S. Schneeweiss, S. Setoguchi, A. Brookhart, C. Dormuth, P. S. Wang, Risk of death associated with the use of conventional versus atypical antipsychotic drugs among elderly patients, CMAJ Feb 2007, 176 (5) 627-632; DOI: 10.1503/cmaj.061250. https://www.cmaj.ca/content/176/5/627. Accessed December 7, 2022.

92   Ventegodt, I. Kandel, J. Merrick The therapeutic value of antipsychotic drugs: A critical analysis of Cochrane meta-analyses of the therapeutic value of anti-psychotic drugs used in Denmark Journal of Alternative Medicine Research ISSN: 1939-5868. Volume 1, Issue 1, pp 63-69 © 2009 Nova Science Publishers, Inc. http://www.livskvalitet.org/pdf/63_240_JAMR_2009_Volume_1_Issue_1_-_FP_Version.pdf. Accessed December 7, 2022.

93   Komossa K, Rummel-Kluge C, Hunger H, Schmid F, Schwarz S, Duggan L, Kissling W, Leucht S Olanzapine versus other atypical antipsychotics for schizophrenia, May 31, 2013. http://www.cochrane.org/CD006654/SCHIZ_olanzapine-versus-other-atypical-antipsychotics-for-schizophrenia. Accessed December 7, 2022.

94   Moncrieff J (2015) Antipsychotic Maintenance Treatment: Time to Rethink? PLoS Med 12(8): e1001861. https://doi.org/10.1371/journal.pmed.1001861. https://journals.plos.org/plosmedicine/article?id=10.1371/journal.pmed.1001861. Accessed December 7, 2022.

U.S. reports several studies suggesting that antipsychotic medications may be less effective for *"the outcomes that matter most to people with serious mental illness: a full return to well-being and a productive place in society."*[95] A seven-year follow up study[96] found that after 7 years the group of patients who discontinued or dramatically reduced the dose of antipsychotic medication showed twice the recovery rate (40.4% vs. 17.6%) when compared with people who continued taking a high maintenance dose of medication.

Even proponents of long-term antipsychotics note that patients who discontinue antipsychotic medication develop immediate problems, including anxiety, agitation and hostility. They claim that discontinuing medication leads to a return of the original problems. However, there is strong evidence[97] that the problems arising with discontinuation reflect withdrawal symptoms and not necessarily the return of the original problem. More gradual tapering off reduces the likelihood of original symptom return or of having symptoms of withdrawal. It is useful to note here that the sudden withdrawal of many drugs often causes problems. Consequently, especially in the case of psychoactive medication, clinicians should recommend gradually tapering off when the treatment period is over. The patient should also be informed about and prepared for the almost inevitable side-effects. The prescription should really be for the drug AND for how to take it AND for all these other effects, including when, why and how to discontinue the medication.

Most family doctors and psychiatrists can provide anecdotes of patients who come in on their own or with their families reporting a single episode of extremely bizarre behavior. The doctor may prescribe a medication and might never see the family or patient again. However, now and then a family member will report that the person did not take the medication and is now fine. This shouldn't be surprising, as studies estimate that between 2%-30% of prescriptions are never filled at the pharmacy and many more are not taken as prescribed.[98] Stories like this abound and it appears that the problems seem to resolve on their own. Doctors also observe that a small number of people go on to exhibit very bizarre behavior after an initial episode, whether or not they take prescribed antipsychotic medication. Perhaps we should call this the '**not**cebo effect' (the effect when one does not take the prescribed medication) to go along with the placebo and nocebo effects!

95   Insel, T., Directors Blog, Antipsychotics: Taking the Long View, August 28, 2013 https://www.ethicalpsychology. com/2013/09/antipsychotics-taking-long-view.html. Accessed August 8, 2015.

96   Underink L, Nieboer RM, Wiersma D, Sytema S, Nienhuis FJ., recovery in remitted first-episode psychosis at 7 years of follow-up of an early dose reduction/discontinuation or maintenance treatment strategy: long-term follow-up of a 2-year randomized clinical trial. JAMA Psychiatry. 2013 Sep;70(9):913-20. doi: 10.1001/jamapsychiatry.2013.19. http://www.ncbi.nlm.nih.gov/pubmed/23824214. Accessed December 7, 2022.

97   Moncrieff J (2015) Antipsychotic Maintenance Treatment: Time to Rethink? PLoS Med 12(8): e1001861 doi: 10.1371/journal.pmed.1001861. http://journals.plos.org/plosmedicine/article?id=10.1371/journal. Accessed December 7, 2022.

98   Park, Yoonyoung ScDa; Yang, Hyuna PhDb; Das, Amar K. MD, PhDa; Yuen-Reed, Gigi PhDc,*. Prescription fill rates for acute and chronic medications in claims-EMR linked data. Medicine 97(44):p e13110. https://journals.lww.com/md-journal/Fulltext/2018/11020/Prescription_fill_rates_for_acute_and_chronic.78.aspx November 2018. Accessed Jan 15, 2024.

Chapter 8: ——— More on Non-Pharmaceutical Interventions

KEYWORDS: Intervention, Nonpharmaceutical, Placebo, Behavior Therapy Rewards and Incentives, Talking Therapies, Mood Disorders, Avoiding Inappropriate Medication, Choosing an Advisor

ABSTRACT: Many nonmedicinal maneuvers described in this chapter successfully influence mental health. We cite many of the techniques that professional therapists (and anyone) can use to influence how other people think, feel and behave. We also recognize that, sometimes, drugs may be appropriate for use as chemical straitjackets or mood-management agents in people who are violent or upset and ignore verbal appeals. In this instance, drugs to subdue or sedate someone can be less harmful than physical restraint. Context helps professionals assess the appropriateness of choices.

Juggling Chainsaws ———

From what we wrote in the last chapter, it might seem that prescribing psychotropics to treat mental health problems is a bit like a doctor's juggling chainsaws – but the injury would be to the patient, not the juggler. We recognize that these pharmaceuticals can be useful, especially in very disturbed or out-of-control patients, but they require careful management and should be avoided if that is possible. In the course of making this clear, we mentioned less noxious alternatives that often help patients and bear little danger. We will focus next on these alternatives, but we recognize that all treatments have limitations and possible harms.

Failing to Intervene on a Timely or Adequate Basis ———

In the case of non-pharmaceutical treatment, one issue is a delay or failure to intervene more radically when someone has a diagnosable metabolic disease. This is one of the great challenges of dealing with mental health issues. Doctors can err by acting precipitously with an intervention, or they can err by not recognizing an addressable danger. There is no perfectly safe approach; real consideration of each unique patient, thoughtful decision-making, planning, monitoring, assessing of progress and communicating are all essential. Piloting a helicopter has been compared to balancing on a beachball. Caring for patients with mental health problems is a lot like this!

As clinicians grapple with the problem of which intervention to use, their patients occasionally suffer unnecessarily when there is a delay in the adoption of an intervention that is worthwhile.

PERSONAL MEDICAL EXPERIENCE

DZ, a psychologist by training and occupation prior to medical education, rarely prescribed psychoactive drugs. Usually, more time consuming, non-pharmacologic interventions were enough even for people who seemed to have severe problems.

However, the usual non-pharmaceutical maneuvers failed for 3 patients, two of whom were in medical families. DZ had shared with them the medical literature about the effectiveness of antidepressants, including research showing that antidepressant medications were not usually effective for mild to moderate depression. When other interventions failed, DZ prescribed antidepressants, which each one claimed were of major benefit.

Presumably, for these patients, earlier pharmacological intervention might have decreased the duration of their distress but there was no way of identifying ahead of time that these individuals would be in the group of people who achieved more benefit than harm. These 3 patients might have benefitted if DZ used less rigorous criteria for prescribing psychoactive drugs. However, the cost would have been that many people treated non-pharmaceutically would have been drugged.

Maneuvers to Change Behavior —

Not understanding why someone appears to be mentally abnormal means not really knowing what is wrong with them. This lack of knowledge of cause only exacerbates the challenge of providing treatment because no solution comes into focus for the clinician. Given the mandate to do no harm, interventions must be designed to capitalize on what the clinician knows about the circumstances and the individual who is seeking advice. Non-drug interventions for mental health are the essence of personalized Medicine. Each person is different and each clinician approaches problems based on personal knowledge, perspicacity, beliefs and experiences. Hence, clinicians may differ in their approaches to mental health problems. One challenge is linking individuals looking for solutions to therapists who have congruent skills, experiences and empathy to deal with that type of individual.

The good news is that there are many therapists of different kinds, a multitude of non-pharmaceutical interventions and many approaches that can influence behavior even if we do not know what is causing it. Many measures, even those unrelated to health care, also improve how we think, feel and behave. They include visiting an amusement park, eating ice cream, playing tennis, being with friends, doing work we love, exercising, eating well and going to the beach.

In everyday life, many people sometimes use legal lifestyle drugs like alcohol, caffeine, nicotine and – legal in some jurisdictions – marijuana to improve how they feel. These substances change feelings and behavior in everybody, as do recreational (and illegal) substances, regardless of their psychological state.

Rewards and Incentives —

In everyday life, people also use words, gestures, sticks and gifts to influence others' behaviors and feelings. Economists and psychologists recognize that people usually behave in ways designed to maximize personal rewards, i.e., their pleasure.

It is not always apparent what will be rewarding in a circumstance, because context and individual likes influence what people find bothersome or pleasurable. For instance, children usually enjoy getting candy, especially if it took little or no effort to get the goodies. However, if the context changes, they might reject the candy.

One example is the Ultimatum Game[99]. This game involves 2 children. One child, the 'Proposer', is given chocolates to share with the other participant in any way the Proposer wishes, called the 'split'. The second child, the 'Decider', gets to choose whether or not to accept the split. If the Decider accepts the suggested split, both children each receive some candy and benefit. However, if the Decider rejects the suggested split

---

99 Wittig, M., Jensen, K., Tomasello, M., Five year olds understand fair as equal in a miniultimatum game, J Exp Child Psychol. 2013 Oct;116(2):324-37. doi: 10.1016/j.jecp.2013.06.004. Epub 2013 Aug 3. https://pubmed.ncbi.nlm.nih.gov/23917161/. Accessed December 7, 2022.

(let's say because the other child would benefit more), both children go candy-free. What is interesting is that most children are initially very happy when they receive any candy. However, when the Proposer suggests an unequal split in favor of the Proposer, most Decider children reject the offer and therefore receive nothing. The candy is rewarding in one circumstance but not in the other – so the perception of unfairness dominates. Recognizing appropriate incentives in the context of a person's life is an essential element of behavior modification.

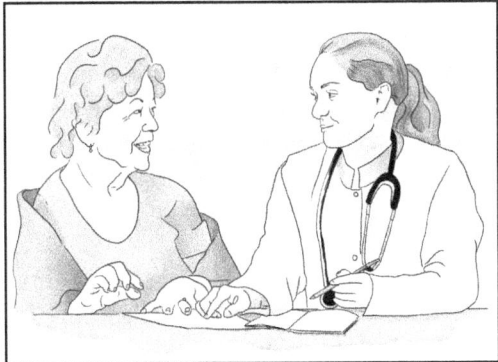

Figure 2.8.1: Talking Can be Effective Therapy!

We mentioned that the terms clinicians use to describe people with mental health problems are often subjective and not applied consistently. Part of the problem is that clinicians may not appreciate the patient's preferences and biases. Sometimes, as we saw in the Ultimatum Game, clinicians are not able to understand the context or the patient's perceptions, with the result that they regard as dysfunctional those behaviors that might be appropriate within the patients' situation and community…they apprehend that any child who would refuse candy must have a mental issue!

Doctors, including psychiatrists, can use simpler and safer interventions that work as well and might be better than other approaches (See FIGURE 2.8.1:

> **Just asking** people to behave in some way is often effective.

> **Incentives** matter: timely rewards and punishment change behavior.

> **Substituting** useful activities for maladaptive ones reduces abnormal behaviors. Going to the gym instead of a tavern leads to reduced alcohol consumption. Chewing gum can substitute for smoking cigarettes.

> **Listening and empathizing**, even though they may be time-consuming, can be effective; just paying attention to someone can help.

> **Engaging** the patient in more formal or structured processes like psychotherapy (which combines all the above) often does help.

Person-specific interventions – think of them as lifestyle prescriptions like a better diet, giving up bad habits and increasing fitness – can also modify how people feel and what they can do. Exercise is especially worthwhile for addressing depression and is a first-line treatment for its milder forms. Most of us are familiar with the benefits of good diet and exercise. They similarly benefit people who may have received mental illness labels.

On the other hand, when these more mundane approaches fail, more dramatic ones may work at least acutely:

> Drugs often reduce agitated behavior and may sometimes be useful for curbing aggressive and violent activity.

> Electro-Convulsive Therapy (ECT) or similar interventions with chemicals can have quite dramatic effects on troublesome memories and behavior. These may, however, injure the brain, and it's difficult to predict ahead of time who will benefit.

> Psychosurgery or brain stimulation change behavior but can go awry (see earlier example of H. M.). The hoped-for results are usually clear, but it is difficult

to make accurate predictions of what the actual benefits will be for a given patient.

The Workhorses of Mental Remedies: Talk·Therapies ———

The more formal or structured methods include 'Talk Therapy', a class of psychotherapies that can be directive or non-directive.

Directive talk therapies, including short-term Cognitive Behavioral Therapy (CBT), focus the patient's attention on specific elements of a problem or on discrete solutions. They are solution oriented.

Non-directive therapies, including Rogerian Therapy, emphasize the strength and capability of individuals to find solutions themselves. Rather than providing directed advice and answers, non-directive therapists create an environment conducive to self-reflection and discovery. Perhaps we should call them 'discovery-oriented'. They help patients to see their issues clearly and then to find solutions within themselves. They do this by asking questions that help the patient to explore and understand issues that gradually emerge from the patient (that is, the problems are 'surfaced' by the patient in response to questions) during the therapeutic encounter.

AN INTERESTING PROGRAM

For fun, the reader can try out Joseph Weizenbaum's program 'Eliza', which is a simple imitation of a Rogerian interaction: https://en.wikipedia.org/wiki/ELIZA. *Despite its simplicity, its author related how people took the program seriously and believed it actually helped them.*[100] *You can try it out yourself.*[101] *When you see how simple it is, you may wonder why they felt that.*

Counselling using non-directive and directive therapies offers effective strategies to reduce depression. "*A review of various treatments for depression including antidepressants, psychotherapy, the combination of psychotherapy and antidepressants, and "alternative" treatments, which included acupuncture and physical exercise found no significant differences between these treatments or within different types of psychotherapy for treatment of depression*".[102]

These Talk Therapies are powerful interventions. Clearly, as the first choice in addressing problems like mild to moderate depression, non-pharmacologic treatments are the most appropriate. Perhaps most importantly, they avoid medication side effects. Consequently, "*If they (drugs) are to be used at all, it should be as a last resort, when depression is extremely severe and all other treatment alternatives have been tried and failed.*"[103]

Perhaps it is most important for all of us to rethink depression. This might involve recognizing day-to-day, mild to moderate (little-d) depression as a common, not necessarily abnormal, occurrence. However, severe (big-D) Depression might demand immediate attention and intervention. Depression at any level is a significant problem that, at its severe level, destroys the enjoyment of life and renders victims unable to function and sometimes suicidal. Here is where pharmaceuticals might have a useful role! It is important to recognize, however, that, even in the case of severe depression, they are not necessarily the first alternative and certainly not the answer on their own.

---

100 Computer Power and Human Reason: From Judgement to Calculation, J. Weizenbaum 1976.

101 http://psych.fullerton.edu/mbirnbaum/psych101/Eliza.htm. Accessed December 7, 2022.

102 Kirsch I. Antidepressants and the Placebo Effect. Z Psychol. 2014;222(3):128–134. doi:10.1027/2151-2604/a000176. https://www.ncbi.nlm.nih.gov/pmc/articles/PMC4172306/. Accessed December 7, 2022.

103 Kirsch I. Antidepressants and the Placebo Effect. Z Psychol. 2014;222(3):128–134. doi:10.1027/2151-2604/a000176. https://www.ncbi.nlm.nih.gov/pmc/articles/PMC4172306/. Accessed December 7, 2022.

Analysis and Treatment of Mood Disorders ⸻

Most people report that they feel sad, tired or lethargic from time-to-time. Some people also report occasions when they are overly energetic and behave inappropriately. For example, they might make expensive and unnecessary purchases, eat or drink gluttonously or suddenly decide to travel to expensive locations, squandering needed resources. Of course, this can go to extremes and be a genuine concern.

Statistics Canada reports that about 7% of Canadians (over 2 million) state that, in the past year, a health professional told them they had a mood disorder, such as depression, bipolar disorder or mania.[104] The American National Institute of Mental Health reports that each year about 10% of people in the United States (over 35 million) report suffering from a mood disorder and that over a lifetime about 20% of Americans will report an episode of mood disturbance.[105] Clearly, there is an issue of definition because almost everyone, including people regarded as "normal", will report episodes ranging from sadness to euphoria over a lifetime.

When a disease, for example diabetes or thyroid disease, causes a mood disorder, the treatment is the treatment of the disease with help for any residual mood problems. Some people, however, who suffer from a mood disorder are labeled as having a 'mental illness' and are called 'mentally ill', even though they lack biomarkers or objective measurements that define a body-based cause of the problem.

Regardless of distress being caused by a disease having no known cause or being an effect of a person's surround, it is important to find a solution! This may be difficult or impossible because many people have serious difficulty gaining access to effective mental health advice. To agree to pay for mental care,

insurance companies in the United States and provincial health insurance in Canada often make the problem worse by insisting that people first get answers from doctors, including psychiatrists. They require this even though other mental health workers are sometimes better and less expensive choices. This just seems dumb!

It also, unfortunately, adds another unique capability to physicians. We have already noted that they have the power of the prescription pad. In addition, physicians seem to have approval authority that empowers insurance companies to pay the fare for care that allied professionals – psychologists, social workers or counselors – will provide. We guess we are fortunate that most mental health problems do not require medications or psychiatrist-specific solutions. Indeed, the overuse of physicians for mental health problems inflates costs, reduces access to care and leads to the unnecessary use of drugs.

It is important to remember that psychotherapists and psychologists use largely harmless conversations as interventions. There are many approaches, as we have documented. Personal trainers can also have a role: they recommend and supervise exercise programs to help people feel more energetic and reduce feelings of depression.

Forestalling Unnecessary Medication ⸻

Treating depressed feelings with antidepressants seems myopic unless these more mundane interventions fail, or the patient has a very serious acute problem requiring immediate intervention. On the other hand, people who lack energy because of a proven biological abnormality do need to see a doctor and to learn what is wrong with their bodies. Determining

104 http://www.statcan.gc.ca/pub/82-625-x/2010002/article/11265-eng.htm. Statistics Canada, Mood Disorders, 2009. Accessed August 11, 2015.

105 National Institute of mental health, any mood disorder among adults, http://www.nimh.nih.gov/health/statistics/prevalence/any-mood-disorder-among-adults.shtml. Accessed August 11, 2015.

that something is wrong isn't a guess or hypothesis – it is finding a definitive cause for the enervation. Doctors must perform comprehensive investigations of people who lack energy or feel depressed. Otherwise, patients risk treatment for mental health problems that don't address the underlying biologic problem. Of course, medical interventions are appropriate to treat the well-defined medical conditions that have associated mental health problems and possibly in the case of severe disturbances.

The conclusion that the flight to drugs is myopic is supported by The Journal of the American Medical Association, which reports that antidepressants are only effective for the small proportion of people who feel severely depressed. The Centers for Disease Control and Prevention reports that 3% of the U.S. population is severely depressed (big-D Depression), while 10 per cent (more than 3 times as many) of the population is taking antidepressant drugs. From 1988 to 2008 there was a 400% increase in the use of antidepressants, now the third most commonly used type of drug in Canada and the United States.[106] This all is a bit scary! It appears that far too many people are on antidepressants. Remember that, for most depressed people, harmless placebos are as effective as potentially harmful antidepressant drugs. In addition, research shows that few benefit from antidepressants.[107] Yet, as we have mentioned, all those who take these powerful agents are at risk of serious complications, including gastrointestinal bleeding and increased risk of suicide and homicide.[108] [109]

This is why safe, non-pharmacologic interventions are where to start even for the acute treatment of severely depressed outpatients.

Better methods are needed to ensure that drugs are prescribed only to those who are likely to benefit. One solution is **only** to refer people with mental health problems to medical professionals after non- pharmaceutical treatments have failed.

It is vital that health services administrators, researchers and health informaticians study the fate of those taking antidepressants. This would deliver crucial data that can serve as ammunition in putting a stop to medication abuse. We need to know if, in the end, pill-takers are more or less likely to have happy and productive lives compared with similar people who decline drug treatment or who try non-pharmaceutical means to alleviate depressed feelings. We do not have, but dearly need, solid answers here.

As diabetes and obesity increase, reports of depression have increased. That is not surprising because the symptoms and behavior (feeling tired, unmotivated, unproductive and lazy) of depressed people are virtually the same as those not physically fit. We will state yet again: improved fitness often leads to improved mood!

Non-Psychoactive Drugs: Anti-inflammatories for Depression —

Sometimes, simpler and safer agents can help in addressing depression.

---

106 Antidepressant Use in Persons Aged 12 and Over: United States, 2005–2008 L. A. Pratt; D. J. Brody. and Q. Gu. NCHS Data Brief No. 76. October 2011. http://www.cdc.gov/nchs/data/databriefs/db76.pdf. Accessed December 7, 2022.

107 Fournier JC, DeRubeis RJ, Hollon SD, et al. Antidepressant Drug Effects and Depression Severity: A Patient-Level Meta-analysis JAMA. 2010;303(1):47-53. doi:10.1001/jama.2009.1943. https://pubmed.ncbi.nlm.nih.gov/20051569/. Accessed December 7, 2022.

108 Fournier JC, DeRubeis RJ, Hollon SD, et al. Antidepressant Drug Effects and Depression Severity: A Patient-Level Meta-analysis. JAMA. 2010;303(1):47-53. doi:10.1001/jama.2009.1943. http://jama.jamanetwork.com/article.aspx?articleid=185157. Accessed December 7, 2022.

109 Coupland C, Hill T, Morriss R, Moore M, Arthur A, Hippisley-Cox J. Antidepressant use and risk of adverse outcomes in people aged 20-64 years: cohort study using a primary care database. BMC Med. 2018 Mar 8;16(1):36. https://www.bmj.com/content/343/bmj.d4551. Accessed December 7, 2022.

Diabetes and obesity are associated with signs of inflammation.[110] [111] [112] [113] This finding and its biomarkers are also associated with other diseases, for example arthritis,[114] [115] which often engender depressed feelings. We do not yet know how inflammation contributes to the feelings of malaise. However, there is evidence suggesting that anti-inflammatories[116] improve depressed feelings and that the change in mood is not related to changes in pain.[117] This may represent an opportunity for research. Perhaps Health Informatics experts and other researchers can determine the characteristics of depressed people whose mood is most likely to benefit from anti-inflammatory medication. Maybe depression associated with diabetes and obesity would be the place to start. No guarantees, but maybe an opportunity to further our understanding!

Choosing a Mental Health Care Provider

In most areas of Medicine, it does not really matter which doctor people choose. For heart disease, thyroid disease, cancers and most conditions with objective biomarkers, most doctors will recommend very similar interventions. For mental health problems, however, people's choice of their clinician often determines if aggressive treatment or if benign interventions will be the starting point. In the latter case, the doctor will see if the problem resolves without imposing the risk of an adverse drug reaction.

Indeed, when referring to clinical practice guidelines, the American Psychiatric Association comments: *"The American Psychiatric Association (APA) Practice Guidelines are not intended to be construed or to serve as a standard of medical care. Standards of medical care are determined on the basis of all clinical data available for an individual patient and are subject to change as scientific knowledge and technology advance and practice patterns evolve. These parameters of practice should be considered guidelines only. Adherence to them will not ensure a successful outcome for every individual, nor should they be interpreted as including all proper methods of care or excluding other acceptable*

---

110 Inflammation as a link between obesity, metabolic syndrome and type 2 diabetes. Esser N, Legrand-Poels S, Piette J, Scheen AJ, Paquot N 2014 Aug;105(2):141-50. doi: 10.1016/j.diabres.2014.04.006. Epub 2014 Apr 13. http://www.ncbi.nlm.nih.gov/pubmed/24798950Diabetes Res Clin Pract. Accessed December 7, 2022.

111 van Greevenbroek MM, Schalkwijk CG, Stehouwer CD. Obesity-associated low-grade inflammation in type 2 diabetes mellitus: causes and consequences. Neth J Med. 2013 May;71(4):174-87. https://pubmed.ncbi.nlm.nih.gov/23723111/

112 V. C Luft, M. I. Schmidt, J. S. Pankow, D. Couper, C. M. Ballantyne, J. H. Young, B. B. Duncan Chronic inflammation role in the obesity-diabetes association: a case-cohort study Diabetol Metab Syndr. 2013 Jun 27;5(1):31. doi: 10.1186/1758-5996-5-31. http://www.dmsjournal.com/content/5/1/31. Accessed December 7, 2022.

113 The inflammation markers used in reference 21 were IL-6, C-reactive protein, orosomucoid, sialic acid, white cell count and fibrinogen.

114 B. A. Hu Saini, S. T. Moore Arthritis Disability, Depression, and Life Satisfaction among Black Elderly People Health Social Work (1990) 15 (4): 253-260 doi:10.1093/hsw/15.4.253. https://pubmed.ncbi.nlm.nih.gov/2276687/. Accessed December 7, 2022.

115 Dickens, C.; McGowan, L.; Clark-Carter, D.; Creed, F., Depression in Rheumatoid Arthritis: A Systematic Review of the Literature With Meta-Analysis Psychosomatic Medicine: January/February 2002 - Volume 64 - Issue 1 - p 52-60. http://journals.lww.com/psychosomaticmedicine/Abstract/2002/01000/Depression_in_Rheumatoid_Arthritis_A_Systematic.8.aspx. Accessed December 7, 2022.

116 Examples of anti-inflammatory drugs include celecoxib, naproxen, and ibuprofen.

117 O. Köhler; M. E. Benros; M. Nordentoft; M. E. Farkouh; R. L. Iyengar; O. Mors; J. Krogh Effect of Anti-inflammatory Treatment on Depression, Depressive Symptoms, and Adverse Effects A Systematic Review and Meta-analysis of Randomized Clinical Trials JAMA Psychiatry. doi:10.1001/jamapsychiatry.2014.1611 Published online October 15, 2014. http://pure.au.dk/portal/files/82334617/JAMA_Psych_Meta_analysis_anti_infl_intervention_depression.pdf. Accessed December 7, 2022.

methods of care aimed at the same results. The ultimate judgment regarding a particular clinical procedure or treatment plan must be made by the psychiatrist in light of the clinical data presented by the patient and the diagnostic and treatment options available."[118] (emphasis ours)

The APA reiterated the intent of this older guideline in a general discussion of guidelines in Psychiatry when they commented "*The ultimate recommendation regarding a particular assessment, clinical procedure, or treatment plan must be made by the psychiatrist* in light of the psychiatric evaluation, other clinical data, and the diagnostic and treatment options available. Such *recommendations should be made in collaboration with the patient and family, whenever possible, and incorporate the patient's personal and sociocultural preferences and values in order to enhance the therapeutic alliance, adherence to treatment, and treatment outcomes.*"[119] (emphasis ours)

In other words, appropriate treatment is up to the individual psychiatrist and the psychiatrist's assessment of the situation and up to the patient to decide whether to accept or reject the advice. Some psychiatrists lean towards at least starting with Talk Therapies, while others prefer an immediate pharmaceutical approach. Given this spectrum of approaches, it is up to patients to ask how often whichever intervention helps or harms people in their circumstances. Health administrators and health informaticians must design and implement information systems that track what happens to people who participate in different interventions. Again, absent data we are left guessing!

An earlier chapter described research by Kirsch and others showing antidepressants, at best, sometimes are better than placebo. Surely, it is logical to initiate care with benign, side effect-free interventions to start patients on the path to mental health recovery, rather than immediately resorting to drugs that in themselves might be harmful.

Summary

Practically every day, we all influence the thoughts, feelings and behavior of those around us for better or worse. We persuade, we listen and empathize, we cajole, we share our experiences, we plead, we reward, and we admonish, as we try to change what people do, how they feel and what they are thinking. Clinical experts use or should use the same tools, even if, from time to time, medications must be added to influence mental health.

---

118 Working Group on Schizophrenia https://ajp.psychiatryonline.org/doi/pdf/10.1176/appi.ajp.2020.177901. Accessed January 12, 2024.

119 Silverman, J., Galanter, M., Jackson-Triche, M, et. Al. The American Psychiatric Association Practice Guidelines for the Psychiatric Evaluation of Adults, Published Online: 1 Aug 2015. https://ajp.psychiatryonline.org/doi/10.1176/appi.ajp.2015.1720501 https://doi.org/10.1176/appi.ajp.2015.1720501. Accessed December 7, 2022.

Chapter 9: ——— Measuring and Categorizing Mental Health

KEYWORDS: Measuring, Outcome Measurements, Benefits of Treatment, Taxonomy of Our Understanding of Mental Health Problems, Thoughts, Feelings, Behavior, Normal Variations, Linking Changes in Mental Health to Interventions, Measures of Mood, Measures of Thought, Measures of Behavior

ABSTRACT: Various scales, some of which are herein, produce measures of mental states – assessments of thoughts, feelings and behavior. Measurement is important because it enables clinicians and researchers to assess and categorize the benefits and harms of various treatments. We discuss the efforts clinicians and researchers use as they attempt to learn more about the natural history of mental health problems and of the influence of various conventional and medicinal interventions.

Why Measuring Mental Health is Important

We want to know about almost everything: Does it work? We ask that about things people try to sell us; we even ask about the health system and the treatment a doctor might apply when it comes to our physical health. What about mental health care? Does it work?

We already know that measuring health[120] – assessing patients' initial health status, the results of the care process and patients' outcome status – is crucial and easily accomplished. Measuring mental health, though, is more challenging.

Understanding how to measure mental health is important because individuals and communities dedicate significant financial and human resources to developing, maintaining, assessing and improving mental health. Unless communities measure the effects of their interventions, they will be unable to assess if they worked or not. Nor will they be able recognize,

retain, improve on, proliferate and apply the most effective services. Attempting to manage in the absence of measurement is, at best, lame.

If researchers and administrators can understand the characteristics of people and their problems and which interventions produce better results, it may be possible to promote the most effective approaches and terminate unhelpful ones. The dearth of data frustrating decisions like this is appalling.

Measuring Mental Health and the Effects of Interventions

In this chapter we describe how we can evaluate mental health before, during and after intervening. We have defined the dimensions of mental health as thoughts, feelings, and behavior. They are the length, width and height of mental space. Interventions in mental health are designed to improve exactly these.

---

120 As a reminder, the dimensions are comfort, function and life expectancy (see chapter on measuring health).

In addition, it is important to recognize that the content and quality of one's social activity and work involvement are important demonstrations of one's mental health. This means that the best measures of mental health will take into account not only discrete elements of behavior – like angry or euphoric outbursts – but also how and how well the person participates in the normal activities of daily life including work, play, rest and relationships.

When patients, clinicians and researchers evaluate the benefits of mental health interventions, they ask if, following intervention, patients had improvements in these dimensions of mental health. Researchers and many clinicians start by applying formal, well-validated, 'instruments'. These are checklists, questionnaires and similar well-tested tools that help the therapist to make formal, structured and carefully documented observations based on specific criteria or measures developed and validated by researchers. Researchers applied these instruments to test subjects and examined how they responded to their questions or other stimuli. These tools are often the product of years of research and validation. This is the way it should be if they are to serve as reasonably objective measures of human emotional, cognitive and functional characteristics and how these are affected by intervention! Though 'reasonably objective', they still have a subjective component, subjectivity sourced both in the patient and the assessor.

Frequently, however, clinicians, like the rest of us, rely on intuitions or seat-of-the-pants sensing to decide if a person is happy or sad, coherent or confused, well-behaved or misbehaving. That is like eyeballing the distance to something in physical space – it is an estimate, and not always a good one, especially since our unaided senses don't perform satisfactorily when it comes to assessing someone else's mental state.

Based on what they think is going on with a patient, therapists choose interventions hoping to help resolve problems, preferably without causing further physical or mental glitches. Therapies also aim, wherever possible, to improve overall comfort and function (including the ability to work and be self-sufficient) especially related to social interactions and self-care.

Detailed evaluation of mental health interventions relies on measures of the change in the quality of thinking and thoughts, feelings and the resultant behaviors. It is not usually possible to detect and measure changes in objective characteristics like we can do with body chemistry or other biomarkers, as there usually are none – at least that we yet know how to detect. Some efforts have been made to assess patients' reactions to interventions using bioelectronic assessments, such as Galvanic Skin Response (GSR), blood pressure, muscle tension and the like. These proxies may give an indication of biologic effects of an intervention but are insufficient on their own to validate changes in mental state.

Our still-primitive understanding of mental health problems, the body's and brain's response to or cause of them and the absence of objective biomarkers, make objective assessment of the impact of care difficult and often impossible. This does not lessen the importance of the patient's problems nor the significance of the therapist's efforts. It also is not intended to devalue patients' and doctors' subjective impressions. It is just that we see the patients' problems and the results of intervention as "through a glass darkly" and we apply far-blunter interventions than typical in physical health care. Given this, our limited knowledge and embryonic evaluation tools make it essential that we encourage and support basic and applied clinical research to develop better approaches to mental health assessment and care. To be truly effective, we must pursue the understanding of the underlying contextual and biological causes of and treatments for mental health problems. Discovering, accurately measuring and understanding the causality and correction of mental health problems is essential for progress. And we still have a long, long way to go.

The reader has learned that some mental health problems reflect well-known and well-understood illnesses. Our examples have included mood disorders associated with thyroid or adrenal disease, as well as thought disorders including hallucinations associated with brain tumors. For mental health problems associated with known diseases with biomarkers, we also have recognized that the treatment is the treatment of the known disease and the assessment of improvement is the change in the disease biomarkers. However, how about the much larger universe of problems absent the knowledge of causes and the existence of objective measures of the effects of treatment?

Categories of Our Understanding of Mental Health Problems

It is worth our while to start with a reminder of our framework for understanding mental health problems and their causes.

TABLE X: MENTAL HEALTH: A TAXONOMY OF OUR UNDERSTANDING OF THE BIOLOGY OF MENTAL DISORDERS

Mental health problems are caused by the following:

1. **A diagnosed medical illness**, *for example, thyroid disease, a brain tumor or a brain development disorder.*

2. **An undiagnosed, elusive, but diagnosable medical illness**

   a. *Some are undiagnosed because the doctor has not considered other possibly rare medical illnesses and has not ordered appropriate investigations.*

   b. *Some are undiagnosed because the condition is very rare, but a suspicious and persistent clinician could search for and eventually diagnose the exact problem (examples include porphyria and hyperparathyroid disease[121]).*

3. **A medical illness that is not diagnosable with current techniques** *because scientific knowledge has not discovered the condition or demonstrated ways to find the disease.*

   a. *Many believe that certain forms of erratic behavior or inappropriate affect represent illnesses that better techniques would enable identification. Examples:*

      i. *some forms of depression, which many speculate represent currently untestable abnormalities of neurotransmitter metabolism, e.g., serotonin.*

      ii. *some forms of behavior labelled as autistic, speculated to be related to genetic brain abnormalities.*

4. **No Physical Illness:** *mental health problems in the context of normal brain and body biology.*

   a. *Learned maladaptive behaviors.*

   b. *Reactions to stress and current social or relationship context.*

5. **Someone else's perceptions or beliefs,** *where someone inappropriately attributes mental health problems to the person.*

   a. *Some children are labelled hyperactive or with attention deficit because a teacher or parent can't answer their questions, is impatient or can't abide their exuberance.*

   b. *An exceptionally thoughtful person who expresses ideas that the other people cannot understand because the ideas are too complex for them or beyond their ken.*

---

121 S. Park and R. Hieber (2016) Acute psychosis secondary to suspected hyperparathyroidism: A case report and literature review. Mental Health Clinician: November 2016, Vol. 6, No. 6, pp. 304-307. https://www.ncbi.nlm.nih.gov/pmc/articles/PMC6007533/. Accessed Dec. 7, 2022.

We went more deeply into this before, but it is worth reiterating about a few of the categories (please refer to the table above).

Regarding the second group of people who have discoverable, but uncommon abnormal biology, unfortunately, absent objective evidence, the clinician may speculate that a patient's problems reflect abnormal biology. Not good! Without knowing which abnormality is involved, this will only be speculation as to a cause and has a high probability of being mistaken.

Related to the third group, one example is the growing amount of data indicating that some mental disorders have genetic correlates. However, because the biological (e.g., gene-based) cause of this category of disorders has not been determined, there are no objective tests clinicians can use to confirm what it is.

The final group includes people who have nothing wrong with them, but people around them are overreacting to or inappropriately judging them and possibly punishing them with pejorative labels. The clinician may have to help the patient (and/or those close to them) find ways to prevent or ameliorate these reactions or to change context to avoid them.

In the absence of biomarkers to identify cause and to assess objectively improvement or worsening of a problem, reliable behavioral and other subjective measurements are crucial. Only through these will we be able to understand if and how well treatments are working. However, a major challenge for clinicians and researchers, which we have discussed, is distinguishing the effect of treatment versus the normal variations in mood, behavior and thinking in response to daily living. Although many ideas in mental health are controversial, few people would dispute that normally, from hour-to-hour and day-to-day, mentally healthy people experience variations in thinking and mood. Sometimes they are happier; sometimes, sadder. Sometimes they have bizarre ideas and sometimes they are just planning a creative romp in the bedroom. They do this normally, unrelated to any mental health problem or intervention.

Measuring Variations in Mental Status – What is 'Normal'?

Measuring normal variations in mental state is interesting and important. When we can recognize normal variations, it will be possible to distinguish normal from abnormal states. However, defining what normal variations are is elusive, a moving feast, and they vary according to culture and time. Measuring changes in mental health following interventions is also essential if we are to determine if treatments are worthwhile. The challenge is to recognize when changes are caused by an intervention or would have occurred naturally or reflect a change in the person's context including the attitudes of friends and neighbors.

Perhaps it is useful to examine the concepts of 'natural' and 'normal'. We would submit that things happen 'naturally' if they are either not affected by people or they are always affected in similar ways by people. In other words, they are not artificial.

We toss around the term 'normal' quite often. Really this term is a transplant from statistics, meaning that our characteristics follow a 'Gaussian' ('Bell Curve') or 'Normal' distribution. This can be applied to things like people's height and weight and other physical characteristics. When applied to behaviors, it is intended to mean essentially that, on average, people tend to behave in a range of ways. The fact is, though, that the Normal distribution has what are called 'tails' at the extremes. Height is a good example: some people are quite short, while others are extraordinarily tall. However, on average, humans tend to have a relatively narrow range of heights in any population – an Asian population being overall shorter and a Tutsi population being overall taller. Given there are no true limits to the upper or lower ends of the distribution, to say someone or something is normal is at best inexact and at worst judgmental or even demeaning of those at the extremes.

TALLEST AND SHORTEST PERSONS

Robert Wadlow was the tallest human documented so far. He was a victim of acromegaly – a disease of the adrenal glands – and was 8 feet 11. 1 inch. https://www.guinnessworldrecords.com/records/hall-of-fame/robert-wadlow-tallest-man-ever

The shortest documented person was Pauline Musters, who measured 21.5 inches. https://en.wikipedia.org/wiki/Pauline_Musters

This is another way of saying that 'normal' is a movable feast. In the case of mental health, 'neuro-typical' might be a better word than 'normal' for behavior that is <u>common</u>. The use of the word 'neuro-typical' tries to sidestep the problems with the word 'normal', which is really a statistical term. 'Neuro-typical' just means that human brains are similar and that we think, feel and behave in ways that are familiar, usual and common. However, we must recognize that there are huge variations.

Measuring mental health is also important because social environments are such a strong influence on how people think, feel and behave. As communities evolve, it is worth knowing how changes in communal behavior influence the mental well-being of community members. For example, does opening a factory improve community well-being because of the benefits of new jobs? Or does the new factory reduce community happiness because it raises expectations regarding the wages at existing companies or is perceived to be polluting?

Remember the dimensions of mental health. Interventions in mental health may improve an element in a specific dimension, for example, the feeling of sadness that had been interfering with overall function. Alternatively, that intervention may also reduce overall function by causing weight gain, decreased activity or changes in libido. For example, doctors might prescribe mental health treatments, like antidepressants, hoping to reduce feelings of depression and improve immediate happiness but instead inflict other problems on the patient. Interventions can help or harm. The important message is that humans are complex entities – their response to intervention can be unexpected or undesirable.

A case in point is marijuana. As it becomes more prevalent, it will be interesting to see its impact on the use of prescribed psychotropic drugs. Will the use of antidepressants increase or decrease? Will people self-medicate? Will marijuana use lead to an increase or decrease in prescriptions for antipsychotic medication? We don't yet know, and it will be difficult to find out due to the nature of human beings – the prescribers, the users and the observers!

Experts worry that legally or illegally secured drugs, which might produce an immediate improvement in happiness, might also have associated high costs from decreased engagement and reduced productivity. Moreover, it is not clear if antidepressant use is associated with increases or decreases in cognitive function or the ability to work – some patients report that antidepressants have undesirable effects even on their desire to participate in sex. The problem is magnified because the effect of both psychotropics including antidepressants and placebos is similar. The psycho-pharmaceutical 'knife' often cuts both ways and sometimes in no important way at all!

Evaluation of Mental Health Interventions Requires Measurement of Changes in the Dimensions of Mental Health <u>and</u> in Overall Function

What is important is that measures of mental health and of the effectiveness of interventions must assess not only the anticipated positive changes, but also the negative influences, such as reduction in overall productivity and engagement in social relationships. Just as we expect hip surgery to improve overall function, not just reduce pain, so we expect mental health interventions to be of overall benefit. The risk is that some interventions in both physical illness and in mental health problems trade-off improvements in one area with decreases in another area, like social interaction.

Eating a poor diet, living in harmful environments and not exercising lead to impairments in physical **and** mental health. *"Mental health and many common mental disorders are shaped by various social, economic, and physical environments operating at different stages of life."*[122] People, who are poor, socially disadvantaged, and have little access to education are more likely to suffer mental health problems. However, not everyone in these categories develops such problems. Similarly, some people who suffer from a traumatic event develop mental health problems that impair their ability to function. Others, having suffered traumatic stress, continue to function well or become stronger. Nietzsche's comment *"what does not kill me makes me stronger"*[123] applies to some people but not to others.

One challenge is to identify those people who are resilient and those people more likely to be incapacitated by traumatic events or poor social environments. Anyone who is interested in this problem must understand how to measure and classify mental health states and problems.

Measures of Mood

Mood is a subjective state of mind or feeling. It is what we sense of our own emotional state. There are at least 7 emotional states: anger, fear, disgust, happiness, sadness, surprise and contempt.[124]. Generally, what we mean by "being in a good mood" is that we are happy and are not feeling any of those other emotions.

Most of us know how we feel. Clinical efforts to assess and influence mood therefore rely on patients' reporting of their own moods, that is, the patients' stating they feel cheerful, sad or other emotions. What is more, mood and behavior are related. People in a good mood say that they feel like being active and enthusiastic; those in a bad mood, that they are sluggish and tired and would rather disengage. In addition, body cues, including facial expressions, also influence care providers' impressions of the mood of the people. If a person's affect (say, a sad look) does not conform with statements of being happy, that tells the provider that something is awry and that the person likely needs attention. Lack of congruence between statements and displayed affect (sometimes called 'inappropriate affect') is an indicator we all use in judging social situations. Displayed affect is a 'tell' (like in poker) that, if incongruent, causes suspicion about the patient's statements. It may also indicate that the patient is trying to hide or mask something. The eyes have been called the "window of the soul", but it's really the whole face that can circumvent conscious attempts to not show emotions. The good news is that humans are quite good at reading faces, but sometimes they are fooled by them, a skill of conmen.

NLP

There is a pseudo-science called Neuro-Linguistic Programming (NLP) that makes far more of our facial expressions and gaze than scientific evidence has or probably would be able to validate. It claims, for instance, that the direction of gaze of a person's eyes indicates the person's 'brainedness' – if they are more analytical (they associate that with a dominant left brain and right handedness) or synthetical (they associate that with the right brain and left handedness). The only value DC has derived from it are the observations of the detrimental effects of inappropriate affect when speaking. It can be awful when a person gives sad news while exhibiting a smile, or positive comments with a sad or angry

122 World Health Organization Social Determinants of Mental Health. WHO and the Calouste Gulbenkian Foundation May 14, 2014 https://www.who.int/publications/i/item/9789241506809. Accessed Jan 15, 2024.
123 German: "Was mich nicht umbringt macht mich starker."
124 https://en.m.wikipedia.org/wiki/Mood_(psychology). Accessed February 10, 2023.

face. In particular, it was very revealing to DC when friends told him during conversations that he did not look like he was listening or that he did not smile when he claimed to be happy. NLP was created by Richard Bandler and John Grinder in the 1970s in California, U.S. and has been used to provide psychotherapy – even though it has no valid basis.[125] [126]

People, in being introspective, use a variety of self-assessment tools to identify, analyze, assess the appropriateness of and track their own feelings. They might examine how a change in their situation leads to changes in mood and can memorialize this to help them to recognize mood changes.

FIGURE 2.9.1 below describes the characteristics of mood. On the vertical axis, it shows at the top and bottom that we can feel activated or deactivated. On the horizontal axis, the sides show that our feelings can be pleasant or unpleasant. Words for activated-pleasant states include excitement and elation. Words for activated-unpleasant states include 'tense', 'angry', and 'upset'. Alternatively, we can feel deactivated. Descriptors for deactivated-pleasant states include 'relaxed', 'calm' or 'content', while descriptors for deactivated-unpleasant states include 'sad', 'depressed', 'bored' or 'fatigued'.

These methods of identifying and classifying feelings are used in therapeutic environments. They give the therapist a window into the patient's mind and feelings. Furthermore, the therapist may ask the patient to record feelings and the situation in which they occur in a diary or on a smart phone. Both the therapist and the patient can review those notes retroactively, perhaps discovering associations and noting the temporality. Anyone can use this when facing depression and even for noticing that one is getting better or worse.

The idea here is that humans are bundles of emotions, and the emotions in which we

are wrapped at any given time vastly affect our mood and, thus, our sense of contentment and psychic balance. Mood is where many, if not most, therapeutic interventions first focus.

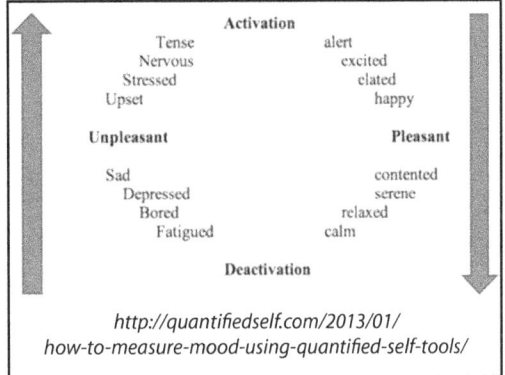

http://quantifiedself.com/2013/01/how-to-measure-mood-using-quantified-self-tools/

FIGURE 2.9.1: Self Mood Measures

Measures of Behavior

Scream and yell or smash your desk while in the office and others (and maybe even you) will notice and be concerned. Behavior is how we exhibit or act out our feelings and thoughts. It is how the emotional rubber hits the social road, so to speak.

Clinicians and researchers use observations and measures of behavior to learn about how we function, what we may be thinking and feeling and how we affect both those around us and ourselves. Therapists can also use behaviors to determine which interventions might be most effective if altering undesirable behavior is necessary. In order for it to be amenable to research and useful for clinical care, we must measure behavior objectively.

If someone engages in repetitive, apparently compulsive activities – like walking in one direction, then turning around and going in the opposite direction, then repeating again and again – it is possible to measure the amount of

125 J. Sturt, S. Ali, W. Robertson, D. Metcalfe, A. Grove, C. Bourne, C. Bridle Neurolinguistic programming: a systematic review of the effects on health outcomes. British Journal of General Practice 2012; 62 (604): e757-e764. DOI: 10.3399/bjgp12X65828. https://bjgp.org/content/62/604/e757. Accessed Dec. 7, 2022.
126 https://en.wikipedia.org/wiki/Neuro-linguistic_programming. Accessed Feb. 10, 2023.

time they spend on the activity and determine if it interferes with accomplishing their goals. In the case of other behaviors, such as repetitive handwashing, the behavior may provide insights into the person's thinking and feelings, like an irrational fear of germs or contaminants. It may even provide a direction for intervention, like the need to reduce fear.

Of course, we have to recognize that some behaviors clinicians regard as peculiar, some communities may consider normal, while others may not. Acceptable behaviors are those that people and their communities accept as contextually appropriate. Therefore, deciding that a certain behavior is a sign of a mental health abnormality might depend on community values and what the tolerance is for deviation from community norms. For instance, in religious communities, people might regard a person who skips church as bizarre. In atheistic communities, the person who frequents church might be perceived as abnormal and suffering from a delusion.

Usually, communities accept behavior that is outside their norm if it does not harm or annoy others too much. On the other hand, a community might class a behavior as deviant if it is unusual there. They might even regard it as a sign of a mental health problem or even a mental illness if it is unacceptable to them.

A Consequence: Mental Health Diagnoses are Moveable Feasts —

In previous versions of the Psychiatric Diagnostic and Statistical Manual used by psychiatrists to guide diagnosis, experts regarded homosexuality as a form of mental illness. Now it is not identified as such and experts and many communities accept homosexuality as an acceptable variation within a normal range of behaviors. Suddenly, homosexuality is no longer seen as a mental illness or a sign thereof. However, some cultures continue to regard homosexuality as a deviation, immoral or illegal. In some, homosexuals can be imprisoned or even executed. The conventions of the day and the tolerance of friends and neighbors to behaviors have profound influence on what people regard as signifying a mental health problem.

Psychometrists (experts who administer and interpret psychological tests) have a choice of many highly structured and tested questionnaires to measure and report on human behavior. An excellent book, Measuring Health: A Guide to Rating Scales and Questionnaires,[127] reports on several questionnaires used to measure and assess social health and social behavior. Most of these questionnaires recognize that people are social beings and evaluate not only individuals' behaviors and activities but also relationships with the people around them. That seems highly appropriate!

Rating scales are better than intuitive assessments of behavior, because they usually include some quantitative estimate of function that is reproducible over time and in the hands of different professionals. When people use intuition to assess behavior, their judgement of a person's behavior and how it changes is also a reflection of the observer's mood and attitude at the time. Consequently, intuitive judgements might not be reproducible. Therefore, one person's claim that someone's behavior is odd might not be consistent with a neighbor's impression of the same behavior. The mental state of observers significantly affects their evaluation of people when it is based on intuitive judgements. The observers' experiences, emotions, biases and context all come into play. It is not good to have a rubber ruler in carpentry or in mental health assessment!

The value of behavior rating scales is that they are reproducible. When people hear that an expert has applied a certain psychiatric label to an individual, it is important to ask which specific behaviors the individual displayed or

---

127 Ian MacDowell, Measuring Health: A guide to rating scales and questionnaires (3rd edn) Oxford Press. https:// academic.oup.com/book/27457. Accessed December 7, 2022.

reported that led to the psychiatric diagnosis. It is also important to understand the criteria the expert used to conclude something. It can be argued that the definition of an 'expert' should include that the person can provide a factual and rational basis for any statements, as well as being able to specify and substantiate any criteria applied to arrive at a conclusion.

TIMES HAVE CHANGED

Years ago, DZ reviewed psychiatric certificates at a Canadian mental hospital. Psychiatric certificates were papers completed by a psychiatrist that justified involuntary detention in a mental hospital. One certificate reported under "Evidence Justifying Involuntary Detention" that "this woman does not like housework". Clearly the times and values have changed!

Measures of Thinking ————

Thought disorders are associated with false beliefs, also known as 'delusions' often associated with illogical or flawed thinking. In almost all circumstances, developing a worthwhile conclusion depends on there being demonstrably correct beliefs or premises and on clear and structured logical processing from those as a basis. We all need to operate differently from the psychiatrist who completed the certificate in the anecdote above!

Thought disorders are rare. About 2% of the population will, over a lifetime, report a thought or belief that clinicians might consider as seriously abnormal.[128] On the other hand, using the Psychosis Screening Questionnaire,[129] about 4% of the population report having thoughts that might reflect disordered thinking.[130] However, most people who have an occasional disordered thought pattern do not suffer adversely as a result.

Context is important. Just as the context determines whether behavior is regarded as normal or as abnormal, so also does that context influence the interpretation of the person's thinking.

Some beliefs, which may not be correct, are common in certain communities. We all know that many religious people hold strong beliefs that are not compatible with the beliefs of non-believers or believers from other religions. We must conclude that that many people have "incorrect" beliefs, so called delusions – albeit as judged relative to others with different beliefs – yet we do not consider those people as having mental health problems. Their beliefs may be compatible with those of other people with whom they associate. They are not false for them and their community of choice! We simply have no way of knowing which are, in fact, the holders of false or true beliefs when it comes to religion, politics or other ideation held in common within certain groups. What is interesting is that it probably does not matter unless one group tries to interfere with the beliefs of another group. As we suggested, a delusion is only truly significant if it influences how people think about themselves or relate to the people around them.

Thinking is also subjective. No one can definitively describe what anyone else is thinking about or considering at any moment. We can get a rough idea of what we think they

128 Kessler RC, McGonagle KA, Zhao S, Nelson CB, Hughes M, Eshleman S, Wittchen H, Kendler KS. Lifetime and 12-Month Prevalence of DSM-III-R Psychiatric Disorders in the United States Results from the National Comorbidity Survey. Arch Gen Psychiatry. 1994;51(1):8-19. doi:10.1001/archpsyc.1994.03950010008002. https://pubmed.ncbi.nlm.nih.gov/8279933/. Accessed December 7, 2022.

129 Bebbington, P.E., and Nayani, T., The Psychosis Screening Questionnaire, International Journal of Methods in Psychiatric Research 5(1):11-19 April 1995. https://www.researchgate.net/publication/232432002_The_Psychosis_Screening_Questionnaire. Accessed December 7, 2022.

130 N. J. Wiles, S. Zammit, P. Bebbington, N. Singleton, H. Meltzer, G. Lewis Self-reported psychotic symptoms in the general population, The British Journal of Psychiatry Jun 2006, 188 (6) 519-526; DOI: 10.1192/bjp.bp.105.012179. http://bjp.rcpsych.org/content/188/6/519.full. Accessed December 7, 2022.

are thinking – that is called having a 'Theory of Mind',[131] [132] a feeling that we know what the other person thinks or believes – and we often use that when we interact with people. Consequently, people rely on statements from the individual and on perceptions of certain types of behavior that result from their thinking. As we touched on above, one can get some sense of what another person is thinking from facial expressions and other 'body language' – police use this a lot when attempting to detect lies or guilt. However, despite their training, they are not always right. Unfortunately, it may be very difficult for people with personality disorders or serious autism to form a theory of mind of another, making it difficult for them to interrelate with others. Having a theory of mind is not at all the same, however, as definitively knowing what a person is thinking. Rather, we are just able to get a vague sense that helps us discern their 'drift.'

Speech is the most obvious manifestation of thinking, and clinicians can produce objective measures of speech patterns. Examples of disordered speech include:

Flight of ideas – when someone leaps from topic to topic, breaking a logical thread in a conversation.

Blocking – when someone inappropriately or inexplicably frequently stops mid-sentence.

Tangential thinking – when the person does not stay on topic and seldom returns to the topic.

Perseveration – when the person continues focusing on a topic, repeating words and ideas (sometimes despite even having had a response), even though it is clear that the other parties in the conversation want to change topic.

Neologisms – when the person makes up new words, known only to himself (the authors may be guilty of this and Shakespeare is noted for it).

Incoherent answers – when the answer is unrelated to the question or not at all understandable by listeners. However, the role of context is important. Politicians and communications experts, as part of media training, may be taught to avoid a direct statement on a topic or provide a 'talking point', even though it is unrelated or unresponsive to the interviewer's questions.

Echolalia (echoing another person's speech) – for example when someone says, "Do you feel tired?", the responder answers with "Do you feel tired?" Again, context is important. In Rogerian therapy, the therapists might repeat the patient's comment in the form of a question to encourage the patient to find solutions to a problem. Many therapists believe that this is a useful therapeutic strategy, and it seems to work in circumstances where it is important to encourage someone to respond.

Reporting hallucinations – seeing, hearing, smelling, tasting or feeling things that are not objectively observable by others.

Reporting or acting out delusions – sometimes, these are delusions of grandeur: claiming to be the king or queen or claiming to be God, Jesus or a child of God.

Other behavioral manifestations of thought disorders include inappropriate dress for the circumstances (of course, we must discount the fact that men are accused of this disorder by a significant other virtually every time they go out) or failure to maintain even minimal expectations of good hygiene.

To understand and develop interventions for thought disorders, it is necessary to use objective measures of the behaviors that people, including clinicians, regard as abnormal. Then it is necessary to measure the changes in behavior and thinking achieved by interventions. However, it is not just the behavior itself. To understand mental health problems, clinicians, researchers and the public must be able to identify and measure the

---

131 https://iep.utm.edu/theomind/. Accessed Feb. 10, 2023.
132 https://www.simplypsychology.org/theory-of-mind.html. Accessed Feb. 10, 2023.

significance and deleterious impacts of the specific unusual thoughts, feelings and behaviors that pose problems.[133]

Generally, mental health workers are not trying to control or cure an identifiable disease, but rather to modify abnormal thinking, abnormal behavior and abnormal emotions.

SOME RESOURCES FOR MEASUREMENT:

https://ps.psychiatryonline.org/doi/10.1176/appi. ps.56.3.273. Accessed Aug 13, 2023.

https://cpr.bu.edu/resources/. Accessed Aug 13, 2023.

https://www.psychiatry.org/psychiatrists/practice/ quality-improvement/. Accessed Aug 13, 2023.

---

133 https://en.wikipedia.org/wiki/Thought_disorder. Accessed Feb 10, 2023.

Chapter 10: ———— The Diagnostic and Statistical Manual (DSM)

KEYWORDS: DSM, Diagnostic and Statistical Manual, Why Catalog of Mental Health Problems, Labelling, Problems with Mental Health Labelling, Labelling as an Illness, Depression

ABSTRACT: The DSM (Diagnostic and Statistical Manual, in many versions, currently DSM-5) is an effort by mental health professionals to categorize mental problems. Many of the labels in DSM are vague (they are mainly statements of nebulous symptoms) and difficult to distinguish from one another. One consequence is that clinicians often disagree about which label is most appropriate for a client. Some mental health professionals also mistakenly think that a descriptive label of a problem defines the problem's cause. For example, when patients complain they feel depressed and the doctor says they have 'Depression', it is as if this is similar to saying they have 'measles', a disease caused by a virus. In this latter instance, the label 'measles' has value, as its cause is known. Those who 'diagnose' the cause of a mental problem through the use of descriptive labels (where a cause is not known or is unsure) mislead themselves and their clients into believing there is an understanding of the biological cause for the patients' feeling depressed.

Manuals, Manuals and Manuals —

Every profession develops libraries that document the key concepts related to their domain. If you have ever visited a lawyer, you probably saw an impressive array of tomes on shelves that fill the walls of meeting rooms. These, because of the nature of legal work, usually contain the laws and the previous decisions that can serve as the precedents to help lawyers to decide on an approach that might serve a new client. Civil Engineers also have their libraries, often filled with books addressing different types of structures and the strengths of various materials. Even your local mechanic will have resources like this to help in the diagnosis of what's wrong with your car's engine. Every physician has access to material that can be inspected either during a patient encounter or at a quiet time later. The only difference today is that these medical information resources are less frequently seen by clients and patients because they are online or in the 'cloud'. But they are vast!

Physicians' libraries, wherever they reside, explain the causality of disease and help the physician determine a linkage between a patient's symptoms, signs and findings and their cause. Psychiatrists are physicians who focus on mental health, an area, as we have seen, where identifying causality is often difficult or impossible no matter how vast the psychiatrist's library is. Psychiatry is often the realm of the subjective. Usually, self-reported symptoms and therapist's perceptions are its legal tender. Images like 'pinning jelly on a wall' and 'corralling clouds' come to mind. Yes, there are some instances where symptoms and the therapist's perceptions can be tracked back to 'concrete' causes but that may be the exception, not the rule.

Psychiatrists committed to bringing greater certainty to the profession have made a long journey in attempting to create far-clearer statements of the different kinds of mental health problems, how to identify them, what they indicate and what to do about them. Some of this work has been embodied in a sequence of tomes: The Diagnostic and Statistical Manual of Mental Disorders, shown in FIGURE 2.10.1, is now in its fifth incarnation (DSM-5 or DSM-V, using the Roman numeral).[134] Maybe it was predictable, given the subject, but many find it underwhelming…though it is the B+O (Best and Only) of its kind. Despite its nature, it is worth our while to consider it.

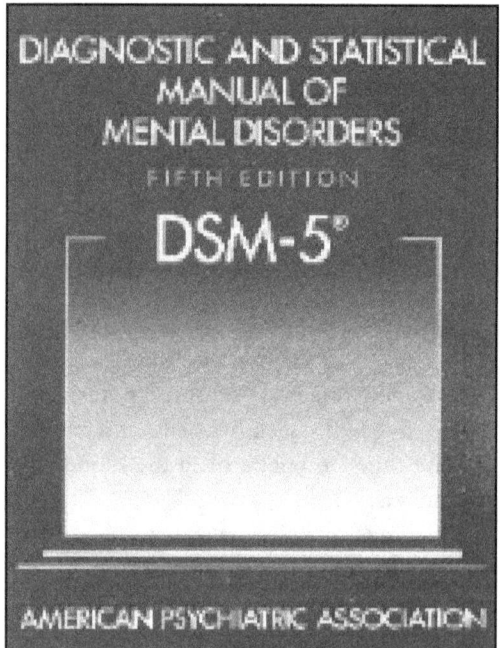

FIGURE 2.10.1: The DSM-5 Manual

Rationale for DSM

Mental health researchers and clinicians have tried over many years to develop a consensus information resource for psychiatric diagnosis and terminology in the form of a manual that could help them assign diagnostic labels to people with mental health problems. The original purpose was to develop a classification system to support research by identifying groups of people with similar mental problems and defining which interventions are most likely to help. This is a standard scientific approach. In Medicine, grouping together people with similar symptoms and findings makes it possible to understand what the common factors causing them are and to determine a specific cause. Once the cause is known, then the physician can hypothesize that patients with similar characteristics will share the same cause and can verify that via further testing. This has been done in Internal Medicine, creating tools like the International Classification of Diseases Tenth Revision, Clinical Modification (ICD-10-CM)[135] and ICD-11[136] and the Systematized Nomenclature of Medicine - Clinical Terms (SNOMED-CT).[137] As might be expected, creating a classification tool for mental health diagnoses has proved to be even more challenging than for Physical Medicine.

The Problems of DSM

Unfortunately, the most recent version of DSM-5 leaves a lot to be desired, notwithstanding the enormous, multi-year and dedicated effort of many thoughtful people to develop it. One of the greatest problems has been dealing with the fact that there are large

134 American Psychiatric Association. (2013). Diagnostic and statistical manual of mental disorders (5th ed.). Washington, DC: Publisher. Text citation: American Psychiatric Association, 2013. https://psycnet.apa.org/record/2013-14907-000. Accessed Jen 15, 2024.

135 https://www.cdc.gov/nchs/icd/icd10.htm. Accessed Feb 10, 2023.

136 https://www.who.int/news/item/18-06-2018-who-releases-new-international-classification-of-diseases-(icd-11). Accessed Feb 10, 2023.

137 http://www.snomed.org/. Accessed Feb 10, 2023.

variations among patients and some with different characteristics will receive the same label, while those with similar characteristics will receive different labels. Additionally, as we have mentioned, community context influences our mood, thinking and behavior and it affects therapists' labelling activity. People with the same label can come from different contexts and may actually be different despite their other similarities. They may have different biological or other causes for their problems. Treatments for mental health problems, as for many other disorders, are influenced by the patient's – and the therapist's – context. Just as the treatment for bowel disorder must consider the diets of different cultures, so the treatment of mental health problems must recognize the influence of community context. However, consideration of community context is mostly absent from DSM-5.

A workaround that some mental health workers prefer is giving prose descriptions of a patient's mental problems, avoiding the labels. They focus on the presenting problems and their treatment. Elsewhere in this section, we have discussed the categories of interventions that mental health workers and others use to influence mental status.

The original developers of the DSM decided which constellations of problems deserve their own descriptive labels. However, there are often no objective biomarkers on which the clinician can base the choice of label.

Creating something like the DSM is inherently challenging. The main difficulty for those attempting to create a nosology or classification system for mental health problems is that we do not have a sufficiently sophisticated understanding of the mind. Creating diagnostic labels for physical illness is hard enough, even though we believe we know the causes, which body systems are involved, what is wrong with them, which symptoms and signs we should

expect and how to go about (e.g., with testing) demonstrating or proving that is what is happening. We still have a long way to go to do that with the brain and our mind.

Transforming Normal to Abnormal

Critics of the DSM categorization complain that some of the labels make normal problems seem like mental <u>diseases</u>. The result is that the apparent incidence of mental illness appears to be increasing. But this may be because of the vague labels. It is just too easy now to label almost everyone! We must appreciate that more people than ever before are being labelled mentally ill even though there is no evidence of an increase in aberrant behavior in the community.[138]

Dr. Allan Frances argues that the DSM-5 categorization is poorly conceived and increases the risk that clinicians will prescribe inappropriate medication by treating the label, not the person. He suggests, for example, that the label 'Disruptive Mood Dysregulation Disorder' will turn ordinary temper tantrums into a mental disorder, justifying inappropriate medication as a first choice, rather than recommending behavioral and educational interventions.[139] [140] Maybe we should consider 'labelling' to be a disease!

LABELLING CAN BE A DISEASE!

People suffering from a variety of impairments may take steps to have the person they are shine out past whatever disability they have. Being labelled as blind or deaf can dramatically affect how others treat a person. One consequence is that those affected take many steps to draw more attention to their personhood rather than their problem and accomplishing that can be hindered by the label. People who are blind are discouraged from 'clicking', which allows a properly skilled person to echolocate objects and

138 https://www.sciencemag.org/news/2010/02/new-criteria-psychiatric-diagnoses-proposed. Accessed Feb 10, 2023.
139 https://www.psychotherapy.net/interview/allen-frances-interview. Accessed Feb 10, 2023.
140 https://science.sciencemag.org/content/327/5972/1437. Accessed Feb 10, 2023.

avoid obstacles in their environment. However, clicking would let others know they are blind! One doctoral student that DC advised developed a silent sonar device that allowed people to do this without drawing attention to themselves. Some of us (perhaps the nerds) don't suffer from our labels, but, for others, labels deny people privacy, independence, equity or effectiveness. Remember that we label someone a 'kook' to dismiss them and what they are purveying.

A somewhat sadder negative effect of labelling was experienced by a physician at an institution for which DC provided consulting services. In this instance the physician had a terminal brain tumor and was devastated when colleagues began to ignore him. He was labelled with 'dying' and, therefore, of lesser at least long-term value.

Users of the DSM-5 classification might also conclude that the exhibition of normal grief is a 'Major Depressive Disorder'. The consequence of that is that sufferers could end up ingesting pills, instead of internalizing the consolation that comes from family and friends and the *"gradual acceptance of the limitations of life"*.[141]

Another example further illustrates the issue. The label 'Asperger's Syndrome' (now incorporated into 'Autism Spectrum Disorder') applies to people whom a clinician believes have difficulty understanding the emotional displays and perspectives of other people. These individuals might not engage in socially acceptable ways and might exhibit a set of repetitive behaviors. Some of our colleagues have described some people as having Asperger's Syndrome, although others thought the descriptors "quirky", "insightful" and "academic" were more appropriate. Normality, brilliance and eccentricity are in the eye of the beholder! Most people, including doctors, do not have special skills or the broad experience necessary to recognize the full range of normal behavior. However, they more often agree with

the judgment of mental illness when people display extreme mental health aberrations, such as is the case with severe autism.

If we are not thoughtful and careful with labels – especially those that can stigmatize – we can willy-nilly do damage to people. People who are shy and avoid some types of group activities used to be regarded as normal. Now, the DSM-5 enables us to label them as having 'Avoidant Personality Disorder'. Both the co-authors of this book seem to slip into and out of that disturbing disorder based on the day of the week, our moods, our workload and the makeup of crowds we endure…and that endure us.

"Another way that the increased prevalence of mental illness occurs is by lowering the threshold of what it takes to be diagnosed with a given disorder. For instance, DSM-5 changed the criteria for "generalized anxiety disorder," a disorder that involves excessive and persistent worrying. Whereas the criteria in DSM-IV [DSM-4] required three out of six symptoms of worrying, only one symptom is needed in DSM-5. Similarly, whereas in DSM-IV the symptoms must have persisted for at least six months, in DSM-5 the duration has been reduced to three months. So, if you are excessively worried for three months about your finances or your health or that of a family member (to the point where you can't control the worries), you would be considered to have a disorder, whereas in the past you would not have." [142]

A PERSONAL EXPERIENCE WITH LABELS

DC was raised a Catholic, though there is no indication of that today. His mother was very devoted and highly observant. One day decades ago, the Catholic Church in its wisdom declared that denying oneself meat on Fridays was no longer obligatory. In Mother's mind, not eating meat on Friday was a

141 https://www.psychologytoday.com/us/blog/dsm5-in-distress. Accessed Feb 10, 2023.

142 Abnormal Is the New Normal, Why will half of the U.S. population have a diagnosable mental disorder? R S. RG, April 12, 2013. https://slate.com/technology/2013/04/diagnostic-and-statistical-manual-fifth-edition-why-will-half-the-u-s-population-have-a-mental-illness.html. Accessed December 7, 2022.

duty and an emblem of Catholicism and violating this mandate was thought to be written in the Great Book as a soul-damning mortal sin punishable by an eternity in Hell. She went through a time of great philosophical dislocation when this requirement was ablated. She once said that she could not understand why it was that one week a person would go to Hell for eating meat on Friday, while another week that was okay. It seems in retrospect that avoiding meat on Friday was a symbol to her of her Catholicism and its absence demanded radical treatment: replace the Pope! The same thing bothered millions of people when Latin was replaced by the vernacular in the Mass. Labels are important!

An Example: Depression ———

The same criticism applies to the label "depression".

The table below designates 9 problems associated with depression according to DSM-5. To receive the diagnosis, a person must demonstrate at least 5 of the 9 problems. The reality is that people with one set of 5 symptoms might be very different from those with a different set of 5 symptoms. Using a single category to describe people who have very different symptom-constellations makes it difficult to organize rigorous research and define thoughtful treatments. Further, if it turns out that there is a biological basis for depression, it is <u>not</u> likely that those having a very different set of symptoms will indicate the same or different biological dysfunction.

The reader can easily see that the categorization of problems in DSM makes research difficult, because an intervention that is appropriate for one group with specific symptoms, to whom the label is correctly applied, might not be appropriate for another group with a different set of symptoms and either group might or might not have the label correctly applied.

A consequence of calling the reactions, like depression, to everyday living a 'mental illness' is that people get ascribed what amounts to a medical diagnosis, and medical intervention becomes the preferred solution. Critics note that a large proportion of the panel that created the DSM-5 catalogue have financial ties to big pharma. Perhaps they are merely afflicted with the dread disorder 'Hypergraphia'…the compulsion to write, or 'Povertyophobia' and want to ensure a healthy cashflow. Ok. That may be unfair. Over the years before DSM-5 was published, there were many expressions of concern in the literature and this is definitely a challenging domain. Perhaps that was the best that could be done…if something actually had to be done.

However, Mental Health Problems are Important! ———

Mental health problems are real and sometimes serious – they may interfere with the enjoyment of life and daily function. Some mental health problems may even lead to suicide or murder. However, it is almost impossible to predict people who are most likely to commit suicide and "*risk categorization may be of limited value or worse potentially harmful, confusing clinical thinking*".[143] It is also important to realize that many antidepressants are associated with increased, perhaps doubled, risk of suicide.

Regardless of the terminology people use to name mental health problems, we must develop and evaluate interventions intended to improve mental health. It is hard to understand, however, if DSM-5 has the potential to serve as a useful tool for research and evaluation. Nonetheless, it or a successor version may be able to provide at least some basis for evaluating the selection and outcomes of mental health treatments.

143 Roger Mulder, Giles Newton-Howes, Jeremy W. Coid. The futility of risk prediction in psychiatry The British Journal of Psychiatry Oct 2016, 209 (4) 271-272; DOI: 10.1192/bjp.bp.116.184960. https://pubmed.ncbi.nlm.nih.gov/27698212/. Accessed December 7, 2022.

FROM DSM-5[144]

Conditions Required for the Diagnosis of 'Major Depressive Disorder'

In order to understand the challenge of applying a diagnostic process in the case of mental health, it is useful to look at the approach used in DSM-5 related to depression.

In order to call a problem 'Depression' using the DSM-5 criteria, five (or more) of the following symptoms must have been present during the same 2-week period and represent a change from previous functioning. At least one of the symptoms must be either (1) "Depressed mood...", or (2) "Markedly diminished interest or pleasure...".

Note: *Do not include symptoms that are clearly attributable to another medical condition.*

1. *Depressed mood most of the day, nearly every day, as indicated by either subjective report (e.g., feels sad, empty, hopeless) or observation made by others (e.g., appears tearful).*
2. *Markedly diminished interest or pleasure in all, or almost all, activities most of the day, nearly every day (as indicated by either subjective account or observation.)*
3. *Significant weight loss when not dieting or having weight gain (e.g., a change of more than 5% of body weight in a month or decrease or increase in appetite nearly every day.*
4. *Insomnia or hypersomnia nearly every day.*
5. *Psychomotor agitation or retardation nearly every day (observable by others, not merely subjective feelings of restlessness or being slowed down).*
6. *Fatigue or loss of energy nearly every day.*
7. *Feelings of worthlessness or excessive or inappropriate guilt (which may be delusional) nearly every day (not merely self-reproach or guilt about being sick).*
8. *Diminished ability to think or concentrate, or indecisiveness, nearly every day (either by subjective account or as observed by others).*
9. *Recurrent thoughts of death (not just fear of dying), recurrent suicidal ideation without a specific plan, or a suicide attempt or a specific plan for committing suicide.*

In addition:

A. The symptoms must cause clinically significant distress or impairment in social, occupational, or other important areas of functioning.

B. The episode is not attributable to the physiological effects of a substance or to another medical condition.

The presence of at least 5 of the 9 criteria, when combined Items A and B, indicates a major depressive episode.

Note: *Responses to a significant loss (e.g., bereavement, financial ruin, losses from a natural disaster, a serious medical illness or disability) may include the feelings of intense sadness, rumination about the loss, insomnia, poor appetite and weight loss noted in the 9 criteria, which may resemble a depressive episode and result in that psychiatric diagnosis.*

Although such normal reactions may be understandable or considered appropriate to the loss, the presence of a major true depressive episode in addition to the normal response to a significant loss should also be carefully considered. This decision inevitably requires the exercise of clinical judgment based on the individual's history and the cultural norms for the expression of distress in the contest of loss.

The occurrence of the major depressive episode is not better explained by schizoaffective disorder, schizophrenia, schizophreniform disorder, delusional disorder, or other specified and unspecified schizophrenia spectrum and other psychotic disorders.

There has never been a manic episode or a hypomanic episode.

144 American Psychiatric Association. (2013). Introduction. In Diagnostic and statistical manual of mental disorders (5th ed.). Washington, DC: Author. http://dx.doi.org/10.1176/appi.books.9780890425596. Introduction.

Chapter 11: —————— Predicting and Treating Dangerousness

KEYWORDS: Predicting Danger, Mens Rea (Latin; law meaning: 'guilty mind'), Art of Medicine, False Positive Determination of Danger, False Negative Determination of Danger, Doctors as Judge and Jury, Psychosis, Drug Benefit and Risk, Murder, Psychic Psychiatry, Violence

ABSTRACT: The dream of mental health professionals and criminologists is to develop tools that help predict if a criminal will reoffend, if an ordinary person is dangerous, or if someone who committed a crime is likely to reoffend. Unfortunately, there are no such tools, and mental health professionals have means no different from those used by lay people to predict dangerousness – and neither group possesses those magic tools. Age, type of crime and criminal history do help predict the chance of a person repeating an offence, but there isn't much else. Indeed, judges and lay jurors, most of whom lack a mental health background, are often asked to mediate between the conflicting opinions of psychiatrists or other "experts" arguing either for the prosecution or for the defense. Jurors' opinions – that's, at least for now, the best we can do!

Introduction ——————

Bombings, shootings, stabbings and beatings are all inflicted by people – dangerous people! Why is it that we almost never know who they are until they do a dastardly deed?

The answer to this question is that we have a particularly daunting problem in identifying the likelihood of someone's being a danger to self or others. Every community has experienced incidents where a person, previously regarded as normal, suddenly became violent and harmed others. The hope, sometimes a fervent belief, is that trained individuals, mental health workers or law enforcement personnel will be able to detect who is likely to become dangerous. Further, we hope someone will be able to intervene early enough. History shows that this hope is forlorn.

Communities also expect that trained professionals will have the skills to understand the state of mind of people when they committed violent crimes. Prosecutors and defense lawyers rely on the concept of *"mens rea"* (Latin; law meaning: 'guilty mind'), a person's state of mind or intention to do something one knows is wrong. If the defense can prove that the person did not know right from wrong or what the consequences of a behavior would be, the court cannot find the person legally guilty of a crime. Perhaps even more pertinent, we might believe that knowing the person's state of mind would enable us to recognize an incipient threat. We all dream, sometimes while not asleep!

This chapter discusses the information anyone might use to predict future mindfulness. It will look at some of the ideas that graduates of medical schools or of mental health training programs use to identify potentially harmful individuals. Armed with such ideas, they might be able to prevent harm. We must emphasize, however, that we are not aware of any scientific (or merely reliable) method that permits accurate and non-contentious assessment of another person's 'state of mind'. If there were objective and measurable criteria beyond those that most lay people use to decide if someone is capable or incapable of understanding right from wrong or of murdering, then any knowledgeable person could apply those criteria. In the absence of scientifically validated criteria, all of us and our courts must rely on conflicting opinions, proffered by counsel or by defense and prosecution 'expert' witnesses, that juries then somehow judge.

Predicting Dangerousness ———

Despite the lack of objective criteria, the police, courts, friends, relatives and other community members often call on doctors and other mental health workers to assess if an individual is likely to harm self or others. We assume that they expect these professionals to somehow apply the 'art' of Medicine, as there is no evidence-based method for doing so.[145][146] Police usually, in fact, will not intervene related to a mental health problem unless the person has already harmed someone or made a credible threat to do so.

TO BE CLEAR

Fear not! All is not lost. Although mental health professionals are not better at predicting dangerousness than the general public, some individual characteristics have been shown to contribute to more accurate predictions of future violence.

The good news is that the most useful predictors involve information that is available to everyone in the community. We all will have some ideas about how to identify people who are likely to be dangerous and those likely to be safe. Common and readily available heuristics or 'rules of thumb' permit communities to recognize people likely to be dangerous and common law generally supports legal incarceration of those who are most likely to be dangerous in the future.

"Readily available clinical information allowed the prediction of assault over 2 years, in a sample of general psychiatric patients with psychosis, with a level of predictive accuracy comparable to that described using more detailed risk assessment tools. The information used in the predictive model was age, sex, having committed an assault in the last 2 years (self-report) and having used any drug in the last year (self-report)."[147]

A medical degree does not confer the specialized skills to assess the evidence to determine if a person will commit a violent offence in the future. If there are objective, scientific, predictors of future violence, then anyone who knows the evidence will be able to apply it in a particular circumstance. If the determination is not scientific, there is no reason to expect that any specific kind of professional will make better predictions. Doctors are no more able than lawyers, judges, or police to assess the evidence and reach a conclusion.

'Experts', in the face of uncertainty, aggressively suggest locking people up.[148] The issue of false positives again rears its ugly head!

---

145 J. Bonta, J. Blais, H. A. Wilson, The Prediction of Risk for Mentally Disordered Offenders: A Quantitative Synthesis 2013. https://www.publicsafety.gc.ca/cnt/rsrcs/pblctns/prdctn-rsk-mntlly-dsrdrd/prdctn-rsk-mntlly-dsrdrd-eng.pdf. Accessed August 8, 2015.

146 Farnham, F., James, D., Dangerousness and dangerousness law, The Lancet, Volume 358, Issue 9297, 8 December 2001, Pages 1976. https://pubmed.ncbi.nlm.nih.gov/11747914/. Accessed Jan 15, 2024.

147 Wootton L, Buchanan A, Leese M, Tyrer P, Burns T, Creed F, Fahy T, Walsh E. Violence in psychosis: estimating the predictive validity of readily accessible clinical information in a community sample. Schizophr Res. 2008 Apr;101(1-3):176-84. https://www.sciencedirect.com/science/article/abs/pii/S0920996408000480. Accessed December 8, 2022.

148 Wootton, L, Buchanana, A., Leese, M. et. Al., Violence in psychosis: Estimating the predictive validity of readily accessible clinical information in a community sample, Schizophrenia Research, Volume 101, Issues 1–3, April

Furthermore, law enforcement may put doctors into a difficult role. if a person is already known to have committed a violent and illegal action, police or prosecutors might ask a doctor to opine on the chances the person will likely perpetrate another offense. They also might seek advice about incarcerating a person in jail versus in a mental health facility to prevent recurrence. Sometimes, the courts ask doctors to commit a person for assessment (legally require the person to undergo professional assessment) even if there has not yet been a judicial determination of guilt or innocence. At other times, an individual may behave in ways suggesting psychosis, while not having done anything illegal. This may engender a request by officials for clinicians to administer anti-psychotic drugs or sedatives to reduce the likelihood of violent behavior. The question is: are physicians, or anyone else for that matter, able to respond or act with any reasonable assuredness that what they do is appropriate and ethical? After all, intervening this way supersedes the person's rights and prerogatives.

DOCTOR ASKED TO BE JUDGE AND JURY AND DETAIN A PERSON

DZ: In my own practice, a police officer asked me to certify* and enable the commitment of a young patient to a mental hospital. The officer reported that my patient had removed the 'No Parking' bags covering parking meters that were in front of a church. The parking authority had put bags on meters to reserve parking for the funeral of a prominent resident. When the hearse arrived, there was no place to park.

The police officer asked about my patient's condition. Although unsophisticated, my patient was independent and had reasonable mental function. Of course, for reasons of privacy I could not discuss his case with the police or anyone else without permission.

I asked if what my patient had allegedly done was illegal. The police officer said "yes", the man had

committed an illegal action. I said that incarceration in a mental hospital for even a brief period was too long and that the police officer should go through the normal legal channels and charge him. Subsequently, nothing happened, and the man continued his life without, to my knowledge, further contact with the constabulary.

* Certify in this context means preparing a formal document that would enable the police officer to detain the person and take him to a mental hospital for assessment.

Communities ask doctors to predict future violence and to suggest if the bad behavior of someone is jail-worthy or hospital-worthy. Is this a role that we should expect of doctors or anyone else for that matter? To answer that question, it is important that all community members have a fundamental understanding of how clinicians (and we all) make judgements like these.

This is important, as the imposition of a psychiatric label has little meaning (but, potentially, a lot of stigma), at least when it comes to predicting if a person will offend again. Public Safety Canada reports that the recidivism rate for criminal offenders labelled 'mentally ill' is the same as that for offenders not given a psychiatric label.[149] Psychiatric attention does not seem to reduce or increase the likelihood that a person will re-engage in criminal activity.

Clearly, there is a need to intervene when a person is behaving violently. In this case, we need to use all the tools at our disposal. These could include using pharmaceutical agents to pacify a person who is out of control or just upset. However, we need to be careful, as we have often noted that drugs reduce activity. They do this not only related to harmful antisocial behavior but also related to worthwhile activities. That is a real problem. The aim of treatment must be not only to reduce

2008, Pages 176–184. https://pubmed.ncbi.nlm.nih.gov/18302982/. Accessed December 8, 2022.

149 J. Bonta, J. Blais, H. A. Wilson, The Prediction of Risk for Mentally Disordered Offenders: A Quantitative Synthesis 2013.   http://www.publicsafety.gc.ca/cnt/rsrcs/pblctns/prdctn-rsk-mntlly-dsrdrd/index-eng.aspx.   Accessed August 8, 2015.

unacceptable behavior but also to increase worthwhile social and vocational relations. Those latter effects are fundamental to helping a person move away from violence.

The interventions clinicians use to change criminal activity are the same as the ones discussed elsewhere in this section. However, in the case of violent behaviors, communities don't have the luxury of either watchful waiting or a medication trial. Instead, they rely on more dramatic, but not necessarily better, ways of protecting the community by using either incarceration or psychotropic medications or both.

Do Drug Treatments for Psychosis Help or Harm? ————

One way to learn how to achieve better results from pharmaceutical interventions is to follow the fates of fully functional people who receive a psychiatric diagnosis, but who were noncompliant with an initial prescription and yet got better. If we learn their characteristics and what they did on their own, perhaps we can encourage similar people with the same problem to proceed in similar ways. Also, it would be useful and enlightening to follow the fate of medicated individuals in the long term.

This has, in fact, been done, but the result is counter intuitive. Long-term studies show that people are more likely to recover social function if drugs are <u>discontinued early</u>.[150] [151] That is indicative of the challenge of assessing the value of pharmaceuticals. Unfortunately, in the existing studies, full recovery of vocational and social function (about 20% in people who continue to take prescribed medications and 40% in people who discontinued them) is not satisfactory.[152] Moreover, there are reports of loss of brain gray matter (which contains most of the neurons), increased mortality and other health risks.[153] [154] This means that it is important to use the least amount of medication and to discontinue medication whenever the benefits of stopping drugs outweigh or are the same as their direct harm.

QUOTING THE SOURCES

"It is undesirable to expect 100% treatment coverage for depression, given many will remit before access to services is feasible. Data were drawn from consenting wait list and primary-care samples, which potentially over-represented mild-to-moderate cases of depression. Considering reported rates of spontaneous remission, a short untreated period seems defensible for this subpopulation, where judged appropriate by the clinician. Conclusions may not apply to individuals with more severe depression."

150 https://asdresearchinitiative.wordpress.com/2013/08/30/tom-insel-nimh-antipsychotics-taking-the-long-view-the-schizophrenias/. Insel, T., Directors Blog, Antipsychotics: Taking the Long View, August 28, 2013 Accessed August 8, 2015.

151 Underink L, Nieboer RM, Wiersma D, Sytema S, Nienhuis FJ., recovery in remitted first-episode psychosis at 7 years of follow-up of an early dose reduction/discontinuation or maintenance treatment strategy: long-term follow-up of a 2-year randomized clinical trial. JAMA Psychiatry. 2013 Sep;70(9):913-20. doi: 10.1001/jamapsychiatry.2013.1.9. http://www.ncbi.nlm.nih.gov/pubmed/23824214. Accessed December 8, 2022.

152 National Institute for Health and Care Excellence Feb 2014 Modified March 2014, Psychosis and schizophrenia in adults: treatment and management. https://www.nice.org.uk/guidance/cg178/resources/guidance-psychosis-and-schizophrenia-in-adults-treatment-and-management-pdf. Accessed December 8, 2022.

153 Vita, A., De Peri, L., Deste, E., et.al., The Effect of Antipsychotic Treatment on Cortical Gray Matter Changes in Schizophrenia: Does the Class Matter? A Meta-analysis and Meta-regression of Longitudinal Magnetic Resonance Imaging Studies, Biological Psychiatry, VOLUME 78, ISSUE 6, P403-412, Sept. 15, 2015. https://doi.org/10.1016/j.biopsych.2015.02.008. https://www.biologicalpsychiatryjournal.com/article/S0006-3223(15)00099-2/fulltext. Accessed December 8, 2022.

154 Ralph SJ, Espinet AJ. Increased All-Cause Mortality by Antipsychotic Drugs: Updated Review and Meta-Analysis in Dementia and General Mental Health Care. J Alzheimer's Dis Rep. 2018;2(1):1-26. Published 2018 Feb 2. doi:10.3233/ADR-170042. https://www.ncbi.nlm.nih.gov/pmc/articles/PMC6159703/. Accessed December 8, 2022.

"Long-term studies show that people are more likely to recover social function if drugs are discontinued early. However, in the existing studies full recovery of vocational and social function (about 20% in people who continue to take prescribed drugs and 40% in people who discontinued prescribed drugs) is not satisfactory."

Moreover, reports of changes in brain grey matter, increased mortality and other health risks means it is important to use the least amount of medication and to discontinue medication whenever the benefits of stopping outweigh the potential benefits of continuing.[155 156 157 158 159 160]

It is disappointing that we have not been able to find any rigorous scientific studies that track the fate of people who took antipsychotics for only brief periods. This is partly because noncompliant people (those who don't take their medications or, in general, don't follow the therapeutic regimen) are often lost to follow up. There are many confounding anecdotes of previously violent people who complied, behaved socially appropriately, then stopped their medication and performed additional violent behavior. There are also those who stopped medication and had no further problems. Go figure!

Solving the problem of appropriate antipsychotic drug use for dangerous people requires long-term studies to find out what happens to non-compliant people prescribed those medications. Are they better or worse off in the long term? Is the community better or worse off?

COURT ROOM JURY SELECTION

In February 2015, DZ was in a courtroom in San Diego, California observing a jury selection. The short version of the case is that the State accused a young woman of murder for a shooting death that had occurred three years previously.

It was clear that, against a charge of first-degree murder, there would be an insanity plea – innocence by reason of insanity. In California, an insanity defense will be successful if the defense convinces a jury that the accused did not understand the nature and quality of his or her act or was not able to understand the difference between right and wrong. The job of the court and jury, in this instance, would be to determine not only that the accused had done the shooting but also that her frame of mind at the time was criminal.

The activities in the courtroom that day were aimed at choosing a jury acceptable to the prosecution and defense. The jurors completed questionnaires about themselves including information about prior experience, education and attitudes toward expert

155 Whitford, H.A., Harris, M.G., McKeon, G., et. Al. Estimating remission from untreated major depression: a systematic review and meta-analysis. Psychol Med. 2013 Aug;43(8):1569-85. doi: 10.1017/S0033291712001717. Epub 2012 Aug 10. https://www.ncbi.nlm.nih.gov/pubmed/22883473. Accessed December 8, 2022.

156 National Institute for Health and Care Excellence Feb 2014 Modified March 2014, Psychosis and schizophrenia in adults: treatment and management. https://www.nice.org.uk/guidance/cg178/resources/guidance-psychosis-and-schizophrenia-in-adults-treatment-and-management-pdf. Accessed December 8, 2022.

157 Dusi N, Barlati S, Vita A, Brambilla P. Brain Structural Effects of Antidepressant Treatment in Major Depression. Curr Neuropharmacol. 2015;13(4):458-65. https://www.ncbi.nlm.nih.gov/pmc/articles/PMC4790407/. Accessed December 8, 2022.

158 Liu J, Xu X, Luo Q, et al. Brain grey matter volume alterations associated with antidepressant response in major depressive disorder. Sci Rep. 2017;7(1):10464. Published 2017 Sep 5. doi:10.1038/s41598-017-10676-5. https://www.ncbi.nlm.nih.gov/pmc/articles/PMC5585337/. Accessed December 8, 2022.

159 Coupland C, Hill T, Morriss R, Moore M, Arthur A, Hippisley-Cox J. Antidepressant use and risk of adverse outcomes in people aged 20-64 years: cohort study using a primary care database. BMC Med. 2018 Mar 8;16(1):36. doi: 10.1186/s12916-018-1022-x. https://www.ncbi.nlm.nih.gov/pubmed/29514662. Accessed December 8, 2022.

160 Maslej M, M, Bolker B, M, Russell M, J, Eaton K, Durisko Z, Hollon S, D, Swanson G, M, Thomson Jr. J, A, Mulsant B, H, Andrews P, W: The Mortality and Myocardial Effects of Antidepressants Are Moderated by Preexisting Cardiovascular Disease: A Meta-Analysis. Psychother Psychosom 2017; 86:268-282. doi: 10.1159/000477940. https://www.karger.com/Article/Abstract/477940. Accessed December 8, 2022.

witnesses, the law and police. Lawyers for both sides reviewed the questionnaires prior to questioning each prospective juror to determine suitability for jury duty.

During questioning, the defense lawyer asked one young man: "Your questionnaire reports that you believe that the idea of an expert witness is farcical. Do you still hold that belief?" The gentleman smiled and said: "There is no way that anyone can know what a person's state of mind was three years ago". The lawyer said: "But the prosecution and defense will each have experts explaining their beliefs". To this, the prospect answered: "That is the point". The lawyer retorted: "You don't have to accept the opinion of either expert. In a trial, you are the one who will choose between the different expert opinions and decide the person's state of mind". The pros-pect answered, "That's the point; I have no way of knowing and neither does anyone else".

Isn't it odd that courts recognize that lay judges and juries are considered to be able to mediate when psychiatric experts disagree? We do not expect lay people to decide when cardiologists or neurologists disagree. Perhaps that is the point. When experts rely on objec-tive evidence and objective biomarkers of disease, they usually agree or, if they dis-agree, they can point to an objective basis for their disagreement.

Wisely, the prospective juror in the anec-dote above had identified one of the reasons that there is so much contradictory opinion produced when multiple psychiatrists opine about anyone's state of mind.

It must be clear to all of us that no one can really divine what someone else is thinking at any particular time. In particular, there is no formal training that enables us to transmogrify into mind readers. If behavior is completely

irrational (or at least we perceive it as so…after all, what is 'irrational'? by whose standards? Conspiracy theorists may judge that nonbe-lievers are irrational!), many of us excuse that because, in our own minds, we believe the person is suffering from a mental disorder and is not able to understand right from wrong or the consequences of the behavior.

Witnesses, including psychiatrists accepted as experts, implicitly claim not only to have special knowledge about a person's state of mind, but also to have the abilities of seers to predict whether or not people are likely to be a danger to themselves or others.

Most of us recognize that the most impor-tant predictor of violence is a history of vio-lence. We recognize that current tools (unless you believe that the movie 'Minority Report' is not fantasy[161]) are insufficient to intervene in the case of someone suspected of violent predilections. In the absence of a history of actions that are physically dangerous or threats to commit an illegal and violent act, we lack any objective basis for such predictions. On the other hand, can we be sure that a previously violent person cannot recuperate?

The good news is that, in this case, the medical literature and lay insights are in full agreement: Forecasting of dangerousness "… *remains like that of the weather – accurate over a few days, but impotent to state longer term outcomes with any certainty*" and "*Would-be clairvoyants engaged in this form of assessment exercise will make use of "tools" in the form of actuarially-based checklists, which give spurious scientific value to estimations that perform less well than chance.*"[162 163 164]

Not only are 'experts' unable to predict dangerousness better than other people; they

161 https://www.imdb.com/title/tt0181689/. Accessed Feb. 10, 2023.

162 Zitner, D., Collins, The Limits of Psychiatry in the Criminal Justice System, National Post, June 10 2015. https://nationalpost.com/opinion/zitner-collins-the-limits-of-psychiatry-in-the-criminal-justice-system. Accessed December 8, 2022.

163 Farnham, F.R., and James, D.V., The Lancet, Letters, Vol 358. December 8, 2001.

164 Szasz T, Psychiatry and the control of dangerousness: on the apotropaic function of the term "mental illness" Journal of Medical Ethics 2003;29:227-230. https://jme.bmj.com/content/29/4/227. Accessed December 8, 2022.

are also no better at predicting who is safe. It stimulates great consternation that the primitive methods in current use identify many people as dangerous who are safe and identify many people as safe, who later are dangerous. Another test with abysmal specificity and sensitivity!

If experts had and used objective tools to predict dangerousness, it would not be necessary to rely on experts (except maybe an expert in applying a complicated tool). The normal rules of evidence could determine if a person met or would meet the objective criteria of dangerousness. But, to make sure it is clear: **there are yet no such tools**. If psychiatric opinions of dangerousness are not based on science, then the concept of 'expert' is not appropriate. Rather, anyone, including legal experts familiar with the rules of evidence, should be able to opine. There is more about experts in the chapter on Expertise in Volume 3.

Is It at All Possible to Predict Dangerousness? In the absence of true science for predicting dangerousness, the best we can achieve is a kind of statistical or experiential estimation of what might avail. Professionals, who have assessed many individuals and who are knowledgeable about their long-term behaviors, could offer opinions founded on the matches they perceive between the individual at hand and members of the population assessed in the past. This approach is used in Medicine when there is the absence of a scientifically rigorous method of connecting symptoms to a specific disease or other abnormality. It is called 'Case-Based Reasoning'165 and is dependent on several factors, including having a sufficiently large set of exemplars (typically in a database), details of the characteristics of each case, an accurate label for each and the ability to match a new individual to the exemplars. So, in the absence of established science, we should expect that professionals could demonstrate that a similar methodology has been used as the basis for the opinion. The problem, as courts have noticed, is how to choose between the conflicting opinions of self-proclaimed, credentialed experts when each has experienced many examples.

However, fear not! All is not lost. Although mental health professionals appear to not be better at predicting dangerousness than the general public, some individual characteristics that we pointed out, which anyone can observe, have been shown to contribute to more accurate predictions of future violence.

The fact is that the most useful predictors of future violent behavior are based on information that is available to everyone in the community. We all will have some ideas about who is likely to be dangerous and who is likely to be safe. Common and readily available heuristics or 'rules of thumb' permit communities to recognize people likely to be dangerous and common law generally supports legal incarceration of those who are most likely to be dangerous in the future. For example: *"Readily available clinical information allowed the prediction of assault over 2 years, in a sample of general psychiatric patients with psychosis, with a level of predictive accuracy comparable to that described using more detailed risk assessment tools. The information used in the predictive model was age, sex, having committed an assault in the last 2 years (self-report) and having used any drug in the last year (self-report)."*[166]

It should now be clear, however, that a medical degree does not confer the specialized skills to determine if a person has committed a culpable assault in the past or will commit a violent offence in the future. If there eventually are objective, scientific predictors of future

165 Case-based Medical Informatics, S.V. Pantazi, J.F. Arocha, BMC Medical Decision Making. 2004. https://pubmed.ncbi.nlm.nih.gov/15533257/. Accessed December 8, 2022.

166 Wootton L, Buchanan A, Leese M, et al. Violence in psychosis: estimating the predictive validity of readily accessible clinical information in a community sample. Schizophr Res. 2008;101(1-3): 176-184. doi: 10.1016/j.schres 2007.12.490. https://pubmed.ncbi.nlm.nih.gov/18302982/. Accessed December 8, 2022.

violence, then anyone who knows the rules will be able to apply them in a specific circumstance. If the determination is not scientific, there is no reason to expect that any professional will make better predictions.

Sheer chance and circumstance will determine that 'experts', who, in the face of uncertainty, insistently suggest locking people up, will cause many people to be confined. And because they are locked up, it will not be possible to determine whether or not they would have been dangerous. On the other hand, 'experts' who are more daring and rarely suggest incarceration will likely release some people who go on to commit violent action.

A frustrating reality is that expert witnesses in Psychiatry or other psychosocial disciplines are not able to provide scorecards showing how often their opinions were correct or wrong. Without those score cards, their judgements cannot be evaluated and their claim to be 'expert' is specious.

It is appropriate that juries and judges, not medical folk, make the final determination and accept responsibility for deciding if a violent offender should be locked up or released.

Example: Losing Your Head

Headlines about violence provoke all of us to think about and take firm stands on issues related to crime and punishment and on issues of personal responsibility.

Two recent stories, one in Halifax, Nova Scotia, Canada, and the other in the province of Manitoba, Canada caused many Canadians to ask how communities can protect themselves while behaving in a fair and ethical way towards those who have committed violent crimes.

The story of Vincent Li is well-known. Mr. Li, age 39, was travelling on a Greyhound bus *en route* to Winnipeg, Manitoba. He sat next to 22-year-old Tim McLean. Suddenly and without provocation Mr. Li attacked, killed and decapitated Mr. McLean and ate his flesh. Subsequently, the killer reported that he heard voices telling him to commit the violent murder. The court, listening to psychiatric testimony, found him 'not criminally responsible' and sent him to a mental institution. He was declared an undiagnosed schizophrenic. Many were appalled when, only three years later, a panel said that he could be released from time to time with supervision. Subsequently, the courts gave Mr. Li an 'absolute discharge' and freed him from supervision. He had been placed on medication to suppress his schizophrenia and normalize his behavior. However, there is no legal enforcement to assure he will continue to take that medication.

Those who applaud the decision believe that psychiatric experts are clairvoyant and able to predict if someone previously violent will be violent again. Others are skeptical and believe that the violence of a crime and the limited ability of psychiatrists to predict dangerous behavior mean that people who have been violent should receive ongoing, humane supervision in a secure environment. This can be accomplished in either a hospital or a jail.

At this time, which perspective is correct is up for grabs. Let us suppose that we carefully documented previous cases that captured the nature of the person, the intentions, the circumstances, the crime, the sentence, the treatment, the rehab and long-term behavior. Even with all that, the variability and innate complexity of human beings will frustrate any assuredness that predictions regarding the next case would prove correct. Such is the nature of human beings and human life.

Other Murders

Another story brings home the key point. In Halifax, 32-year-old Raymond Noel Denny brutally murdered a popular gay activist, 49-year-old Raymond Taavel. What outraged members of the community was that the murderer had previously been found 'not criminally responsible' and sent to a psychiatric facility after slitting a dog's throat and uttering threats[167]. The defense lawyer hired after the gay activist's brutal murder said: *"Mr. Denny should not have been granted a one-hour unsupervised leave from the psychiatric facility."*[168] A little late but correct on the face of it!

Except for perhaps a small number of psychiatrists, few of us claim to understand why any individual commits a violent act. Some psychiatrists attribute bizarre behavior to one or another form of mental illness. Other psychiatrists, examining the same facts, often reach a different conclusion.

Consider Jeffrey Dahmer, who lived in Chicago, Illinois. Between 1978 and 1991 he killed 17 young men and sometimes cannibalized their remains.

DR. BERLIN – A DZ CLASSMATE

Dr. Fred Berlin was a thoughtful, interesting and curious classmate of DZ. He and DZ attended graduate school together in the Psychology department at Dalhousie University in Halifax. Subsequently, he (as did DZ) went to medical school and Dr. Berlin undertook specialist training in Psychiatry and was hired by John's Hopkins University where he is having an outstanding career as an expert in sexual dysfunction.

A psychiatrist claiming expertise in sexual behavior, Dr. Fred Berlin, testified that Mr. Dahmer was mentally ill and therefore not criminally responsible. Dr. Berlin suggested that mental illness was the only explanation for Mr. Dahmer's bizarre behavior. Other psychiatrists reached different conclusions. However, the jury found that Jeffrey Dahmer, a cannibalizing murderer, **was** criminally responsible for his behavior and sent him to prison. Shortly after his incarceration, a fellow inmate murdered Mr. Dahmer.

Different professional opinions about the meaning of dangerousness account for the varied outcomes of review panels. Experts differ because there is little objective science behind the ideas they expound about a person's state of mind or the likelihood of committing a violent act.

In the Vince Li beheading case, Dr. Phil Klassen, a forensic psychiatrist and V.P. Medical Affairs for Ontario Shores Mental Health Sciences Centre, in Whitby, Ontario, Canada and an assistant Professor at the University of Toronto, opined: *"Bear in mind that there is a statistical relation between the seriousness of the initial act, in this case quite horrific, and a lower risk of re-offense. In other words, the more gruesome an act in the case of an NCR (not criminally responsible) patient, the more likely it is that it was rooted purely in mental illness rather than being personality or substance abuse driven, and therefore the risk of re-offending is lower."*[169]

The whacky result of this kind of weird thinking is that communities are more likely to excuse offenders whose behavior is extremely violent and peculiar, compared with those who use less violent means to murder. We assume that this seems as strange to you as it does to us.

Is There a Class on Psychic Skills in the Psychiatry Curriculum? ——

We have characterized some psychiatrists' predictions of future violence or of past mental state as 'clairvoyance'. This skill is beyond the capabilities of most of us. Yet, we ask judges and juries to mediate between conflicting psychiatric opinions of a person's dangerousness and state of mind. It is challenging to see the sense in that.

---

167 National Post, April 17, 2012 https://nationalpost.com/news/canada/raymond-taavel-murder. Accessed December 8, 2022.

168 Raymond Taavel Death: Andre Noel Denny, Accused in Killing, Is Prone To Violence, Not Homophobia, Says Lawyer Canadian Press. 04/18/2012.

169 Correspondence from Sean Kavanagh May 18, 2012 a reporter with the CBC reporting on an interview with Dr. Klassen.

For emphasis, it is worth noting again that the forecasting of dangerousness *"remains like that of the weather…"*. Dr. F. Farnham and colleagues, publishing in the prestigious medical journal Lancet, suggest that psychiatric assessments of dangerousness *"perform less well than chance"*.[170]

The lack of agreement among experts on how to predict harmful behavior means that decisions to classify someone as a criminal or as mentally ill depend on the beliefs and intuitions of a group of human beings, not on science. Some members of the group may have been endowed by an authority unknown with the title of 'expert'. Some would not have permitted Raymond Denny to have any unsupervised leave; others would behave similarly to the one that released Mr. Denny and enabled him to commit murder. For any individual who committed a crime, the decision to incarcerate, hospitalize or release into the community often reflects the composition of the group making human and even personal choices, not the application of objective criteria.

What to Do About Violence ———

Criminal and violent behavior will always be with us. That said, communities will want to deal fairly with people who harm others and will also want to protect themselves and others from the consequences of crime and violence.

It would be wonderful if we had the insights or the tools to predict the future of individuals who behaved violently in the past. Despite the absence of valid predictive models, communities must still intervene in fair and humane ways to deal with criminal behavior and to protect themselves.

In order to advance, we need to take some serious steps. In the first place, clear, well-based, fair and transparent legal methods must be used to determine that accused people did, in fact, commit a crime. That is guaranteed by the Law of the Land. We cannot tolerate the situation where, in the absence of legal proof, those with mental health issues (legally responsible or not) are judged guilty when actually innocent of the crimes for which they are accused. This is judgement by label. And it happens far too often! Allowing this inflicts terrible harm on people. Being labelled mentally ill is stigmatic and prejudicial, and mentally dysfunctional people can end up being 'profiled' and incriminated by the labels they receive.

However, once the court has determined that an individual committed the illegal act, the legal system must develop clear, fair and evidence-based methods to decide how to deal with the perpetrator. Should the guilty party go to a jail or to another facility that is better able to provide care and help the person avoid reoffending in the future? Right now, we cannot answer this question cogently. This means that scientists must do research to develop evidence-based methods and society must fund that research. To develop methods of the genre, it is crucial that scientists design and conduct research and follow up on subjects to determine which behavioral evaluation and correction methods are effective and which ones do not produce worthwhile results. This is just like we said related to medical treatments! And, after all, incarceration in a jail or a hospital is a treatment.

What is happening now should be unacceptable! We are putting physicians and other people into the position of doing the impossible: reading minds and prophesying the future. En passant, we are putting perpetrators in the position of being subjected to them! Let's leave mind reading and clairvoyance for the magicians and New Year's prediction wonks! We are all illiterate in that kind of reading!

---

170 Farnham, F., James, D., Dangerousness and dangerousness law, The Lancet, Volume 358, Issue 9297, 8 Dec, 2001. Pages 1976. https://pubmed.ncbi.nlm.nih.gov/11747914/. Accessed December 8, 2022.

Chapter 12: ———— Thinking More About Psychotherapy

KEYWORDS: Psychotherapy, Human Interactionist Therapy, Purposeful Relationships, Therapists, Matching Patients and Therapists

ABSTRACT: When two people converse, jointly trying to solve a mental problem like debilitating sadness after the loss of a spouse, we call it empathy, compassion, caring or concern. If one is a paid mental health professional, we label the discussion as psychotherapy. We pay therapists to listen, empathize and help individuals find solutions and sometimes an understanding of their mental health issues. If people are properly motivated and trained, they may (hopefully) gain a certain discipline or adopt thinking structures that help initiate and sustain an interaction of value to their clients. But there is no special 'tool' they have that others cannot have. It is still a discussion. The only magic is the human magic of caring, empathy, compassion and concern.

Introduction ————————

People call it 'head shrinking'! What actually happens in psychotherapy? Why might it be that it works? Might it be more akin to mind-expansion, than head-shrinking?

Hacking Out a Trail to Clarity ——

While writing this book we have given a given a lot of thought and engaged in many long discussions to attempt to explain and clarify the nature of mental health, mental dysfunction and mental illness. We have written about the differences between disorders or dysfunctions of the mind versus changes in the mind due to physical changes in the body, particularly the brain. We have made it clear that pharmaceuticals and other physical interventions affect the brain and the mind for better or for worse. We have not, however, provided any rationale as to why it is that a person can affect another

person's mental health through human interaction: verbal (or talk) psychotherapy.

In truth, neither of us truly understands, at the deepest level, how the process of psychotherapy works. It is hard to see how a conversation (which is a basic characterization of a psychotherapeutic session) might significantly address how we think, feel and behave but that happens all the time when we try to influence others or others we trust influence us. How might a verbal exchange with a therapist help us to surmount problems of the mind or to offset or correct for actual biological illnesses of the brain, for that matter? Every day, psychotherapists of many different varieties, in many different settings – including online – help millions of people with a broad spectrum of mental problems. In fact, families, clergy, friends and many others have conversations with and help untold millions.

Let us think about what might be going on in a psychotherapeutic encounter. We cannot claim the perfect congruence of this description with reality. However, we hope it provides a feel for what occurs.

Opening the Mind to Another – A Personal Perspective

Suppose I am suffering from depression, anxiety, confusion or terrifying fear – it does not matter which or how severely as long as I am still able to function and propel myself to a care provider. We must emphasize that severe problems can immobilize, render the person unable to function and may even extinguish the will to deal with their problems or with life itself. We will limit ourselves to the more common, less severe, problems faced by most people.

If I seek help for problems like these, already I have taken one important step towards eventual resolution: I have sensed I have a problem and I have sought help. Recognizing that I have a problem is the first and most crucial of step, without which nothing else can happen. Sometimes, I may not be fully convinced I have a problem, but significant others have told me that I do. I seek help because I sense or wonder if I might need it.

If I begin interacting with a therapist, what am I doing?

Well, first I am believing that this other human being may help. This provides at least a modicum of hope, which might be a crucial feeling when I am down and almost out.

A second thing I am doing is trusting, which is the next most crucial step in the whole process. I'm trusting this other person. Then, in a very real sense, I am admitting this person into my mind, my personal 'safe room' and sharing my thoughts. I am opening to an outsider my most private feelings, like that I am having a problem and need help. In doing this, I am allowing myself to be vulnerable. This is an amazing thing to do, even more amazing than undressing in front of another person – realize that this person is a stranger! If I think of my

mind as a room, I am admitting the therapist to see private things I typically do not share with anyone. I'm allowing the person into my mental inner sanctum, a sacred place. That is real trust! It enables everything else. This granting of trust will usually deepen, as will my vulnerability, and the encounter will become more and more intimate as we proceed. Trust and vulnerability are keys I give to the therapist to open me up and to enable my being helped.

Once having admitted the psychotherapist into my mind, I reveal my issues, my thoughts, how I feel about things, my weaknesses and also what I think of as my strengths. The expert therapist will have ways of proceeding by asking questions and following up on what I say to help me get over my possible embarrassment, reticence or fears or that always-lingering bit of distrust or mistrust. Perhaps one way of seeing the therapist is as an 'intelligent mirror' in which I can see myself, see even into myself in a structured way.

I, hopefully, see the therapist as being skilled in helping me to see the true nature of my problems, to understand and surmount my misapprehensions, to appreciate my challenges in opening up and in facing up to my problems and to encourage and help me make what might be significant efforts to overcome them. A therapist of genuine value might provide guidance about how to address my problems using the strengths I have and how to go about finding my own solutions. The therapist might also suggest ways to approach the resolution of problems gradually and sustainably, rather than my always seeing them as immovable mountains or susceptible to a quick fix…there usually isn't one.

Over time, as I will likely interact with the therapist several times, I will share my mind-room repeatedly and will work with the therapist. Both of us together, in a very real sense, will be 'inside' my mind, hopefully helped by deepening trust and openness. With the therapist's guidance, I have the possibility of working step-by-step to resolve my major issues or, at the very least, to recognize that the long-term effort required is something I can deal with and actually carry out, perhaps on my own.

It is interesting that, once the therapist is through, my mind becomes my own again, my privacy returns and my dependence ends. This can be hard on me! I may have come to feel close to this person. I may even have become bound by a degree of affection, and perhaps even a degree of dependence. Much as I admitted the person to my mind, I must now graduate to being on my own, perhaps with memories, but now self-standing.

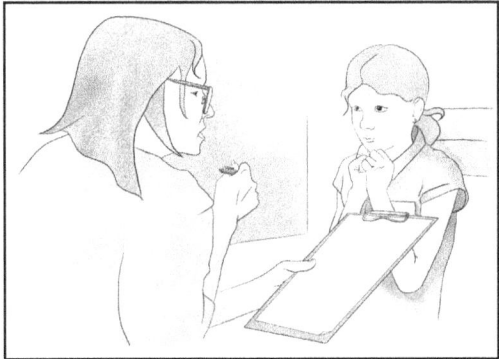

FIGURE 2.12.1: The Importance of Person-to-Person Interaction

Like Other Relationships – But Purposeful (See FIGURE 2.12.1) ——

In reflecting on this process, we recognized that it is not all that different from how any relationship, such as a romantic relationship, forms and progresses. When one feels 'in love', one accepts another person into one's life, overlooks or minimizes the feeling of threat, feels trust and becomes vulnerable. The chemistry of love is a positive one. We seek a partner and closeness and want to continue it. Moreover, in the throes of romantic love, we often ignore or excuse the limitations of the other person. We allow the chemistry and the good feelings to dominate and we fantasize, perhaps, a person greater than reality. We have all been there and

done that! All of this can happen in a therapeutic relationship as well. However, that cannot continue, as the therapeutic partnership is not permanent; it should not exist longer than necessary to resolve my problems.

It is worthwhile to think of the many other kinds of human-to-human relationships and to see the parallels in the therapeutic relationship, including the opportunities for things to go awry. The therapeutic relationship can be so intense that sometimes the therapist falls in love with the patient or the patient is besotted with the therapist. The therapist must have skills to recognize the value of the positive feelings the patient has but always must recognize that this is a therapeutic relationship, not a romantic one. The same is true for the patient. In psychiatry, the process of 'transference' expresses this dynamic. Transference is when the patient 'transfers' onto the therapist feelings that may have been felt for a parent or partner. The patient may develop the feeling of loving the therapist like loving a spouse or a parent. In so doing, the patient may project onto the therapist that those same feelings are shared. This, of course, is rarely the case and, if it were true, the process has gone awry. When the therapist has, for example, erotic feelings for the patient, we call that 'countertransference'.

The nature of the therapeutic process must be the patient's return to absolute independence. The patient must resume normal life, either with the problems resolved or the resolution underway and ongoing. The therapist must recognize that same thing about the patient. Both must go their own ways.

This can be harsh. Even though patients admit therapists into their minds, and even though therapists care for and work intensely and intimately with patients, there must be an end to all therapeutic engagements, a 'casting out', a separation. Both therapists and patients must proceed with their lives! Of course, this leads to areas of great difficulty, and we know of therapists who have not been able to move on, some of whom have been disbarred or even criminally charged. This judgment applies even when patients have fallen in love with them and desperately want a continuing relationship!

ON THE OTHER HAND

In Nova Scotia, a doctor and patient fell in love and eventually married. After they had been married for more than a year, a colleague complained to the College and the doctor had his license suspended for a year. The spouse complained that she would suffer from her husband's loss of income but to no avail. In other professions, people have married parishioners and students. Some would argue that two adults must be free to develop a relationship and that it is presumptuous to prevent professionals from marrying those with whom they work. The problem is compounded for residents of rural communities where there are limited opportunities for doctors and patients to make suitable matches. The main issue is the possibility that the doctor-patient or therapist-patient relationship may engender dependency and this may affect future decisions and freedom. An interesting discussion and debate!

Psychotherapy is an extraordinarily important but intrinsically tricky process because it harnesses our humanity with all its power for the purpose of healing. It is also a risky process because of our foibles. With the kinds of change that need to occur, this should not seem amazing or unusual. There is the saying "no pain; no gain". Taking this risk with a competent and ethical therapist can be – and has been for millions of people – worth it.

AN OVERVIEW OF WHAT THE THERAPIST BRINGS TO THE TABLE (OR COUCH)

- *There really isn't any magic in therapy except the magic of human interaction. Therapy is just good human relations – albeit (hopefully) enhanced by training – in a formal and structured situation. The therapist has invited me into a trusting relationship, and I have accepted. Even this has positive effects.*
- *Typically, the therapist will ask leading questions, such as inquiring as to what is bothering*

me, why I seek help or what form help might take. This shows a desire to help and indicates the therapist's caring.
- *In response to questions, I begin to reveal what's wrong. The therapist has learned about the nature of problems and causes. These questions induce me to go deeper and talk about what I really feel. They cause therapeutic deepening, helping me to explore myself. The therapist can guide me on my journey into myself. Remember "Journey to the Center of the Earth"? This is the "Journey into the Center of Me".*
- *During this time, the therapist actively listens to what I say, providing perceivable reactions. This can stimulate me to say more and what is more meaningful and important to me.*
- *Through the therapist's listening, I may sense that another human being empathizes or even sympathizes with me. This can indicate an understanding of me and my situation.*
- *This questioning, answering and listening provide both verbal and non-verbal exchange, a conversation is occurring, and I can see the therapist understands and appreciates.*
- *In Rogerian therapy the clinician merely acknowledges the patient's comments and prompts the patient to reflect further. Often passive listening and reflection prompt patients to find their own solutions.*
- *This conversation may go on for a long time, over multiple sessions. Sometimes the therapist may have suggestions, strategies or tactics that might help a bit. The therapist can also give some advice or homework, perhaps – although many types of therapists will avoid giving advice, instead eliciting solutions from me.*
- *I can gain from this if I more and more deeply appreciate the real nature of my problems, recognize that they are familiar, realize that there is nothing devastatingly wrong with me and that, perhaps with help, I can climb out of the hole I'm in or at least stop digging.*
- *There are many other possible interventions, all based on the therapist's knowledge of how people think, feel and behave and awareness of the kinds of things that can go awry. This is augmented by skills, like active listening. Further, the therapist can often suggest different approaches to problem resolution, based on knowledge of Human Psychology. One easily understood tactic*

is 'approach-avoidance', where I take baby steps
in to approach something I fear, withdraw and
recover and then approach a bit closer and so on.

A Final Thought ─────────────

Anyway, this is the kind of thing that can happen in psychotherapy. Each person will have a different experience with different therapists. And it isn't unusual to find that a certain therapist just doesn't work for me, necessitating my going to someone else. Similarly, the therapist may find it difficult to help certain patients. A secure therapist will recognize this and possibly refer me to associates or other care providers. Much as I am not perfect, therapists are not perfect and no relationship is perfect.

Psychotherapy is a formal relationship that uses structured methods to achieve outcomes that are the fullest realization of the social power of the human mind!

The next chapter describes some of the formal ideas and methods that therapists use when conversing with clients.

LEARNING TO MANAGE SITUATIONS

Many years ago, while at the university, DC participated in a suicide prevention program. At 3 AM one day, he received a call to come urgently to an apartment where a person was threatening self-harm. On arrival, the person was locked in the bathroom and one could hear pills falling all over the place. The door was locked, so it was promptly broken down and the person brought into the living room. The very agitated individual eventually broke an ashtray and accidentally cut up her hand, drawing lots of blood and stimulating panic. At that point, we called the police. On arrival, they tried to help calm things down. Our joint efforts did not get the situation under control. Finally, one of the officers took DC aside and said: "Let me handle this, ok?" The officer went over to the agitated person and simply said: "If you don't calm down, we will not take you to the hospital!" Amazingly, the person immediately calmed down! DC learned an important lesson that night, which the police had learned from experience: behaviors can be a way of getting what someone wants, rather than targeted on harming oneself.

Chapter 13: ——— Major Varieties of Psychotherapy

KEYWORDS: Psychotherapy, Talk Therapies, Psychodynamic Therapy, Behavior Therapy, Cognitive Behavior Therapy, Rogerian Person-Centered Therapy

ABSTRACT: We discuss several schools of thought related to how the conversations between individuals and professional psychotherapists should proceed. To no one's surprise, opinions differ about the effectiveness of each approach. In fact, a recent book (Treating Psychosis, Nicola Wright, et al.) points out that a therapist may require a cocktail of techniques from many different approaches to deal with some personally-challenging disorders, such as psychotic thinking. For patients, it seems the important issue is finding a person whose knowledge, skills, attitude and behavior are compatible with the person asking for help and advice.

Introduction

There are at least as many flavors of talk therapy or psychotherapy as Baskin Robbins has ice cream and maybe as many as kinds of pickles Heinz claimed it had. Verbal communication is the most common capability humans have to help people or to encourage change to improve their physical or mental health. What we read and what we hear from other people both have important influences on our mood, our resolve to behave in a certain way and our determination to reach desired goals. Conversations with friends, relatives, neighbors and even our own introspection (that 'voice' in my head) influence our view of and response to the world.

The Psychotherapy Conversation

We label conversations as 'psychotherapy' when people pay professionals to converse with them or to give advice on what they might change about themselves and try to learn how they can change. Credentialed talk therapists have studied characteristics and activities of the mind and behavior. Most therapists believe that there are one or more models of therapy that they can apply to help people deal with mental problems.

Therapists usually do not have the luxury of choosing their patients, but patients must decide which type of therapist might best suit them. Consequently, it is worthwhile knowing something about at least a few of the approaches that psychotherapists use.

Unfortunately, we have not found any scientific literature that will help match an individual's characteristics to a type of therapist or to a specific therapist who will most likely help. However, each person might find a type of psychotherapy that is attractive and then choose a therapist who practices it. It is worth noting that this choice is important; each person can benefit from or be negatively affected by psychotherapeutic discussions. Psychotherapy is a powerful intervention!

Kinds of Psychotherapy ———

The major kinds of psychotherapy include the following:

> **Psychodynamic therapies** encourage patients to focus on the inner and hidden workings of their minds to learn which unconscious thoughts and early experiences influence current behavior. The belief behind this is that, with that kind of insight, the patient will be able to overcome obstacles to development and success. Many patients report dramatic and worthwhile change with this method. Others complain that there is no real way to know what hides in the deep recesses of the mind, so the insight the patient develops might be manufactured, prompted by the therapist's statements. In other words, the insights may be like 'false memories' generated, perhaps unintentionally, during the encounter. In any event, we cannot change whatever slights or hurts we experienced in the past, although we might change our interpretation or judgement of them, or we might develop certain strengths that allow us to ignore them. When people think of psychodynamic therapy or psychoanalysis, Freudian Therapy is the first that comes to mind. The Freudian therapist expects the patient to explore relationships with and attachments to parents and significant others.

> **Behavioral therapies** emphasize the role of rewards and punishments in learning new, more adaptive behaviors. There are many who report major successes with behavioral therapy and many studies show the effectiveness of 'systematic desensitization' (we mentioned Approach-Avoidance tactics previously) in helping people to eliminate inappropriate fears. Teachers who give children a time-out in the corner of the room, and parents who send an upset or agitated child to his or her room are using a form of behavioral therapy.

> **Cognitive Behavioral Therapy** is a form of therapy where there is an emphasis on the use of thinking skills in the present to actively change thoughts, mood and behavior. Wikipedia cites: "CBT focuses on challenging and changing unhelpful cognitive distortions (e.g. thoughts, beliefs, and attitudes) and behaviors, improving emotional regulation, and the development of personal coping strategies that target solving current problems."[171] Researchers have demonstrated that this form of therapy is effective for many problems, including depression.

> **Rogerian or Person-Centered Therapy** is a form of talk therapy that encourages patients to reflect on their own lives and come to their own conclusions about what is likely to help the most. In Rogerian therapy (named after Carl Rogers, known as the creator of Clinical Psychology), the therapist reflects back the patient's thoughts, concerns and ideas, seeks reactions and encourages the modification of thinking based on the patient's own values and preferences. Wikipedia describes it: "*Person-centered therapy seeks to facilitate a client's self-actualizing tendency, "an inbuilt proclivity toward growth and fulfillment, via acceptance (unconditional positive regard), therapist congruence (genuineness), and empathic understanding.*"[172]

Different styles of therapies reflect a different emphasis not only on the role of the patient, but also on how determined the therapist and

---

171 https://en.wikipedia.org/wiki/Cognitive_behavioral_therapy. Accessed Feb. 10, 2023.
172 https://en.wikipedia.org/wiki/Person-centered_therapy. Accessed Feb. 10, 2023.

patient are likely to be. Cognitive Behavioral therapies, Behavioral therapies and Rogerian therapies emphasize the here and now and the goals of the patient. They are usually short-term (less than 6 months) and aim to achieve specific well-articulated goals. The psychodynamic therapies encourage people to develop insight into deepest aspects of their mind, a process that might take many years or even a lifetime.

A common feature of all these therapies is that they all require the therapist to be caring, attentive, creative and cooperative with the patient.

Summary

Given the enormous diversity of human interactions, it is no wonder that many varieties of psychotherapies have emerged. The sampling we have provided will give at least a sense of how therapists go about their work. Each approach is based on ideas or theories about how a person can influence and help another. Therapists bring their own history, beliefs and prejudices to their encounters with clients. Somewhere there is likely a person with an approach that is compatible with almost anyone. The main challenge is the one we identified previously: recognizing I am having a problem, deciding to get help and finding the right help for me.

For further reading, we offer the following: https://www.apa.org/topics/therapy/psychotherapy-approaches.aspx. Accessed Feb. 10, 2023.

Chapter 14: ——— There and Care – A Call to Ears

KEYWORDS: Do-It-Yourself Mental Health Interventions, Listening Skills, Human Beings Helping Others

ABSTRACT: Mental health professionals are people too. They suffer from the stresses of their work like anyone else. Sometimes the stories clients tell them are upsetting. Some work excessively long hours because they are committed to serving their community. Mental health professionals, like everyone else, should recognize that their friends, neighbours, and people around them can (and often do) help others and themselves address mental health problems, though some may find it beneficial to get advice from a professional therapist.

The Stress of Professional Life ———

Life isn't a rose garden! Well, unless you consider the thorns!

We have often mentioned that mental health problems are a feature of normal life. It may also be that the best solutions of these problems rest with our friends, family and others that share our lives. What can we each do to help particularly those with whom we work – our workplaces often being sources of stress that affect everyone, some more deeply than others?

The Professional Workplace ———

Most professionals' practices are demanding environments. As the authors are both in the eHealth field, we will reflect on that area, but suggest that anyone can apply these ideas in the context of their own disciplines. This includes those who work in health organizations, as well as the people who work in commercial organizations or academia.

The stresses we all face come at many different points, from many different directions and they are non-stop. Let's consider major electronic systems undertakings, as typical of hospitals. At the beginning of every project, it is essential to select the right applications software, equipment, staffing, plans, staff education programs…the list goes on and on. There is the need to engage everyone in the project, from senior administration to the clinical and clerical staff, plus all those who will implement and support whatever results. Engagement alone, not to mention change management and process reengineering (changing the way people work), can deplete one's energy and sap one's patience. Inadequate engagement and the failure to reengineer work processes in ways suitable to workers are the mortal diseases that have disabled or killed many efforts. Those involved must accomplish everything within a projected budget and timeframe, both of which often suffer from optimism. Slippages in either of those cause the institutional equivalent of major corporal inflammation (a veritable 'cytokine storm' in medical terms). Slippages injure, they hurt, they are urgent problems, the implementors must address them with alacrity, and they can entail the adverse outcome of premature employment mortality.

It's not just that way in healthcare institutions, either. Every company that creates and maintains major software and systems faces deadlines that can wreak terror among staff, and all come with constraints that can cause frustration and the inevitable design flaws and bugs that require immediate fixes. All this occurs against the background of maintaining existing products and somehow ensuring that one's employer looks good every quarter on the stock market if it is a publicly-traded company. A company's survival depends on everyone rowing together and recognizing that the boat can sink.

But You Know This

We are preaching to the choir here. You all know what it's like wherever you sit in whatever industry. It does not matter if you are in senior management or at the mine face of development, implementation, or maintenance. Electronic technologies, for example, have become the analog of electrical utilities with which we move information rather than electrons. The physical and financial health and survival of institutions, clients and patients depend on them. Information is the lifeblood of most, if not all, of today's institutions and the success of technologies and processes that manage this information is depended on by many companies. Electronic systems and software haven't been back-room games for well over 3 decades. It is really important, real time, online, often-on-fire reality in which many find themselves immersed.

Is there any wonder whatever that people submerged in this field (and many others) suffer from mental health problems? In fact, if this were not the case, that would be abnormal. Professionals in high technologies or major utilities would be akin to race car drivers who didn't get scared sometimes, engineers or pilots unflustered by alarms sounding or police remaining stoic when someone points a weapon at them.

This is the important recognition: that many of us, if not all, face intense, daily stress. And that can compromise our mental health. But we must also recognize that society often stigmatizes people perceived as having mental health problems. People may look down upon them, see them as 'different', judge them to be weak and consider them somehow less than they should be. To admit to fears, to depression, to insecurity, to severe insomnia, to feelings of emptiness and meaninglessness, to social and sexual dysfunction, and even to disordered thinking, right up to considering suicide, means we risk social isolation, the loss of 'face', our friends or our jobs. Certainly, in many instances we risk losing the respect of and closeness with those around us. Others may judge and incarcerate us in a private psychosocial fishbowl, quarantined to thwart our contaminating others.

This stands in the face of a reality: that mental health issues are part of the natural human ecology of stressful professions and, for many, they are unavoidable. They may really be a necessary comorbidity of dedication and commitment. Not everyone will have serious mental dislocations, but almost everyone will face at least minor ones. So, we need to help each other, as we illustrate in FIGURE 2.14.1.

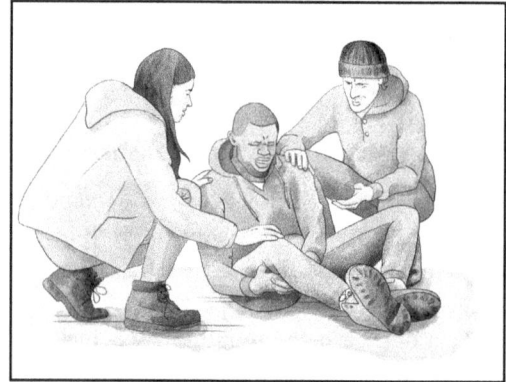

FIGURE 2.14.1: Helping Each Other Supports Our Mental Health

What the Heck Do We Do About This?

In writing about mental health, we have given a great deal of thought to explaining and clarifying what mental health is all about, what can go awry with our minds and what we can do about it. One important concept that emerges from this thinking is that all of us have the capacity and the abilities to deal to some extent with the mental health problems of those around us and ourselves.

It probably goes without saying that to help others, we need to get our s**t (expletive deleted) together. That does not connote that we must be mentally flawless or not have issues ourselves. Even professional care providers have those. Helping others depends on two major things:

1. Recognizing that mental health issues are endemic, universal and the product of the everyday grind and vicissitudes of life itself, amplified in stressful environments.

2. Realizing that there are some relatively simple interventions – think of these as DIY therapies – that we can all apply both to ourselves and to those with whom we have contact.

How We Can Act

Beyond looking at ourselves, recognizing our problems, dealing with them and taking steps that assure and improve our own stability, the next step is to peel our eyes, unclog our ears and pay attention so we notice when others have issues.

When we work with others and rub shoulders with them, we can use **our personal powers of observation and listening skills** to notice if someone has a problem. We can note if someone looks tired and overworked. We can sense if a staff member is upset a lot. We can lend an ear to the scuttlebutt in the organization and take note of others mentioned as facing problems, like financial or relational difficulties. We can **meet with our friends, staff and co-workers and ask how things are going**. And we can make sure that we really hear and internalize their responses. We can **look at their eyes and faces**, not just listen to their words. Or, for some, we can listen carefully to the words despite the expressions on their faces. Expressive and appropriate affect is difficult, filtered or distorted when emotional burdens sit heavily on the mind. We can notice if someone shows signs of a drug or alcohol problem. We can **carefully read our textual communications** from people, remembering the communication via email or instant messaging strips our exchanges of most affect; signs of problems are a bit more difficult to detect in those media. We can **notice the quality of a person's work**, not to judge its excellence but to wonder why it has degraded in any way. Most of all we can be aware, turn up the sensitivity of our 'spider sense' and remember that mental health problems are endemic.

Therapists can become adept at a lot of this sensing, but not all do. However, **there is nothing at all that prevents any of us from becoming better at it**, unless we are lazy or aloof. Human beings have powerful abilities to recognize and 'read' faces! Neurological research indicates that facial recognition is one of the most powerful abilities of the human brain. We all have the fundamental tools, but we have to use them and maybe even hone them for the sake of those around us.

The old declaration that "Mind your own business is the 11th commandment" be damned! **The issues of those around us <u>are</u> our business**, for one thing. Those around us are part of our environment and we depend on them not only for work but also socially and emotionally. We need to care. We must mind them as part of our business!

What Can We do About Others' Mental Issues?

All of us have an amazing set of social skills in our personal tool chests, so to speak. Consider the following:

> **We have a mind and we have ears and we have a mouth.** We can plan to use that mind to think about others; we can ask questions using that mouth and we can listen using those ears. Probably the most powerful tool we have is what we call 'active listening'. This means that we absorb what another person is saying, we think about it and we clearly demonstrate that we are listening, understanding and concerned. Sometimes that's all that people need. How many times has a spouse or partner told you: "You're not listening!" or "You never listen!" The usual excuse is "I was listening" and we have the innate short-term memory capacity to repeat back the last 10 words. But we were <u>not</u> actively listening and were <u>not</u> engaged. Hence the 'F' on the domestic report card! Active listening is a powerful and highly effective step. It will almost certainly improve our grades!

> **We know that human beings can gain simply from the presence of other human beings.** Sometimes, just being with a troubled, lonely or isolated person, sitting together or attending a meeting together while perceptibly connected can make a big difference. Sometimes people just need someone to be there. We may exchange few words, but the sense that someone else is there and – especially when caring is apparent – that can really help. **There and care!** A powerful intervention. Sometimes this is even better than words. Think of how long it takes in a relationship until people can just enjoy each other's presence.

> **We are aware that sometimes others need a little provocation.** We can ask gentle questions, followed by patient silence. The objective is not so much to solicit information (it's not an opportunity to be nosey), but rather to create a space into which the other person can pour out feelings and relieve a crushing backlog. Sometimes gentle questions can lead to a tsunami of bottled-up feelings, bothering or torturing the person. We need the opportunity (the silence and that space) to get that sort of thing out. Listening, active listening, absorbs what is said. Once the person has expressed what is upsetting or troubling, that opens the door to say something or to act in a way that shows empathy, sympathy or concern and a willingness to help, even if that might require someone else's assistance.

> **We have the ability to show others pathways to deeper help.** Beyond the many other ordinary human-to-human interventions we all use without much thought almost every day, there is the possibility of helping someone get additional help. We must handle this offer carefully, as there is usually a reason the person has not done it on his or her own. How we proceed is crucial. It may take another meeting and further discussions. It might even require going with that person to get help or arranging help with the person's permission. This is a sensitive area. If it's handled badly, it can look like we have judged the person as being beyond normal help. But it is normal help! The person may simply need more formal help or more arms-length help if our relationship with them stifles a person's showing certain feelings or blocks revealing potentially embarrassing situations and thoughts. However, if we care, this will not be an unusual step.

The Realities of Mental Health Treatment Today ─────────────

We wrote this because we have recognized that far too many people with ordinary mental issues wait for months for formal therapeutic intervention or suffer quietly in pain and despair. If they do get access to therapists, they might end up medicated, engendering another layer of problems. That may be necessary in the case of someone with serious mental health issues or a physical health issue that causes mental problems. Things like that require dramatic intervention. The focus here, though, is on the more mundane – but still debilitating – difficulties that result from the frictions and setbacks of life and career. If we do encounter more serious challenges, then the ultimate intervention we mentioned above – forwarding to deeper help – is the way to go.

Our contention is that many of our confreres feel marooned and unaided on a bleak mental beach or sent for unnecessarily invasive, costly and drug-oriented professional intervention. This happens although we all have the potential of helping them, of helping each other. We believe that all of us can recognize mental health problems. We do not need to make a formal diagnosis! We can see that these problems are part of everyday life. We can understand they are not stigmata nor are they signs of weakness or disease. We can comprehend and accept that we have a role in helping others with these problems. And we can realize that we can do something significant in helping overcome them.

Whatever else you get out of this chapter, please really be there and really care – there and care. That may make the difference in a person's happiness, peace and survival.

Chapter 15: ——— Further Thoughts on the Nature of Mental Health and Dysfunction

KEYWORDS: Difference Between Illness and Mental Illness, Interventions to Improve Mental Health, Illnesses Influencing Mental Health, Environmental Causes of Mental Health Disturbances

ABSTRACT: The important issues discussed in the section include problems with labelling and problems with recognizing which intervention might be most effective for an individual patient. The chapter reinforces the idea that mental dysfunction can also be a normal reaction to exigencies of a person's context.

Going Over It Once More ———

> **There is a serious problem with the conventional use of the term 'mental illness'!**

We believe that we have made it clear that we see the term 'mental illness' to be a pejorative term, as it implies something physically wrong with the brain (a physical impairment) is causing disturbed thinking, mood or action. For even more consideration of this matter see the Chapter at the end of this section.

Words matter! If we call everyone with a mental problem – a problem of the mind – 'ill', we are putting the entirety of humanity in a box, because no one is without problems of the mind. The designation 'mentally ill' is about as informative as the term 'alive'.

Elsewhere in these books we have mentioned the creation of the term 'pre-diabetic'. That word originated as a marketing label to assist in promotional efforts intended to prevent diabetes. Regretfully, tens or hundreds of millions of people are now more likely to be worried and expending time and money to correct a poorly defined 'problem'. We mentioned that perhaps we should create a new label 'pre-dead' that would apply to an even greater number – all of us – thereby creating an immense marketplace! The solution? Ban that label! That may be the best way to deal with the term 'mental illness', for it would label all of us as candidates for one or other drug or medical intervention! However, rather than killing the term, we will attempt rehabilitation and distinguish between 'mental illness' and 'mental dysfunction'.

True Illness ———

What is an Illness that a 'Mental Illness' Is not?

Illness, as we all know, affects our comfort, how and how well we function and sometimes even how long we live. Illness can cause pain or weakness, for example, and can make it difficult or impossible to carry out the daily functions of life. There are many causes of illness, all of which are physical, which means biological (a virus), chemical (Arsenic) or material (a car impact or a tackle) events cause them. These causes are many – we touch on the types of causes (etiologies) in Volume 1. True illness involves one or more organs of the body or the interactions and transport of substances and signals among these organs.

By calling something a 'mental illness' we are implying that there is something wrong with the body – in this case, something wrong with the brain – that someone can treat by any number of medical interventions, including pharmaceuticals, surgery, nutrition, physical therapy or other physical corrective action.

Illnesses are physical. We need physical interventions or the body's own healing ability to address them. No one can be talked out of a true illness, an aberration of the body's biology (metabolism) or structure. One other way of saying this is that our thinking or feeling cannot correct a true illness. It can make us feel better about the illness, but not reverse it. How we think and behave might, nonetheless, influence those conditions (e.g., like bringing about diabetes by poor eating habits) where better health habits influence our metabolism.

Meditation, positive thinking and prayer can change our mood and how we feel. However, there is no scientific evidence that these elements lead to cures of biological abnormalities. There is, on the other hand, some evidence that people who are religious do tend to live healthier lives. For example, they may smoke and drink less than the people around them. However, there is no objective evidence that people's praying or participating in religious activities will cure any diseases, though many believe this is possible. Belief is not scientific evidence.

ON PRAYER

Years ago, DZ cared for a religious couple. They were thoughtful and polite and always said: "bless you; we're praying for you". Some of their problems related to obesity from reduced exercise and poor eating habits. Usually DZ could persuade, cajole or plead with people to change their habits. This usually

resulted in at least an initial change and weight loss. This outcome is what the research literature reports: the lifestyle changes were not persistent – frustrating for doctors to know. Behavior and dietary changes will improve a patient's health and, for some conditions (hypertension, type 2 diabetes for example), will eliminate the need for medication.

In exasperation, DZ asked the couple if they believed in the power of prayer. They were enthusiastic in expressing their belief in the power of prayer. So, DZ asked them if they thought his prayers for them would help them, even if he were of different religious persuasion. When they said his prayers would be helpful, DZ suggested an experiment. He said he would pray for them to lose weight and track their weight over the following six months. It is delightful to report that offering to pray for them made a big difference. They lost substantial weight over the following six months and maintained their improved health for at least 2 years. This proves yet again that we are each motivated by different things.

Mental Dysfunction

We have used the term 'mental dysfunction' to describe our state when our thinking, feeling or behaviors are problematic. We might not be able to reason clearly or to concentrate. We might not have appropriate emotions, being fearful, for example, of ordinary social conversation or situations. We might not also be able to do certain things and we may show unprovoked rage or violence. These are the dysfunctions of the mind; they are mental dysfunctions.

Illness as a Cause of Mental Dysfunction

Illness can cause some dysfunctions of the mind if it affects the brain in some way. For example, a growth in the brain might cause a person to hear voices that are not real. Diseases of other organs, for example of the thyroid, adrenals or parathyroid, produce changes in our body that influence brain function. A chemical, a common one being alcohol, can dramatically affect how and what we feel and how we function; it can impair our driving, for instance. It is also possible for infectious diseases to invade the brain. For instance, bacteria do this in the case of bacterial encephalitis. The same can be true of viruses and other agents, such as misfolded proteins (prions). Indeed, even the anatomy (the parts and structure) of the brain can be damaged or disrupted by blunt force trauma of the brain that occurs during an accident or an athletic event. In this latter case, blood may collect in a location that puts pressure on or damages parts of the brain. A clot-type stroke is another example; it interrupts normal blood flow to a part of the brain, killing it. All of these affect the structure of the brain and they are all illnesses.

We also must realize that genetic inheritance and early development can cause the child's brain to be abnormal in some way. There is evidence, for example, that genetic mutations can disrupt the normal way that parts of the brain inter-communicate – this is one of the theories of what is behind autism, as we mentioned. Parent's use of drugs and alcohol before or during pregnancy and extremely poor maternal nutrition seem to sometimes cause fetal brain development problems. Genetics (and epigenetics – changes in the expression of genes caused by maternal behavior or environment) and environmental toxins and other factors are among the etiologies of disease. This points out that it is important to review all the possible causes of disease and the effects they have if we are to understand their impacts on the brain.

Mental Dysfunction That's Not an Illness

The challenge is understanding the dysfunction of the mind that does not have a physical basis. This can happen if we experience a circumstance that causes profound or even incapacitating fear. Then, when confronted with a

related circumstance, we feel recurrent terror and are unable to function. Socioeconomic circumstances and our upbringing can also cause mind dysfunction. Our brains are physically normal after facing these circumstances, but our minds can be dysfunctional. There is no physical agent causing that dysfunction; no disease that invaded us or damaged the brain. However, this type of dysfunction is very common and experienced in all our everyday lives. The changes that occur in our brain when we learn something, or adapt to our environment, or react to traumatic stress are normal changes that influence all of us in similar ways. Although our mental function changes in reaction to certain events, our biology has not changed for the worse. The brain does subtly restructure, albeit in an entirely normal way. We will discuss this more deeply below.

Mental Dysfunction that Might or Might Not be An Illness

Some illnesses that influence the brain are rare or difficult to diagnose. It is also likely that researchers have not discovered some illnesses that influence brain biology, and, therefore, currently they are not diagnosable. Other chapters discuss some of these and the consequences that patients face when clinicians treat the mental dysfunctions produced by rare illnesses as if they are dysfunctions of the mind, or are treated based on incomplete, conjectural understandings of what is happening.

There is, Though, a Physical Aspect of Mental Dysfunction

Here is the confusing point. The only thing in us that thinks, learns, feels and manages desired action is our brain. We don't have feelings that are not sourced or remembered in the brain. Likewise, we don't have thoughts that are not based on information (memories) in the brain or where the brain is not doing the thinking. Ditto the control of the function of our body parts, like walking, chewing gum (simultaneously or not) or playing the piano. All these activities are based in and on the brain; they are manifestations of the functioning of the brain, including things like remembering and learning. Of course, physical illness can affect our thinking, feeling, emoting and performing actions (we can feel crappy with a cold, be confused when affected by dementia or be unable to walk because of a broken bone). However, in most cases of mental dysfunction there is no detected physical first cause correctable with a pharmaceutical, surgery, physiotherapy or other biological or physical intervention.

So, we now know that our cogitation, emotions and actions happen in our brains. Beyond that, an important recent insight is that any new thinking, new feeling and new acting change our brains. They change the structure of the brain by forming new neural connections, by altering existing connections among the neurons of the brain or by changing the chemistry of the brain. So, our brains change as we experience life. My brain may start as Brain 1.0 in the womb, become Brain 1.1 on day (or hour or minute) one, progress to Brain version 1.2 on the next day (or hour or minute) and so forth. This development of our brains is a normal event in everyone's life. And this goes on throughout life…subtly restructuring the brain through inter-neuron linkages (synapses). The point is that there are no drugs that can selectively alter these linkages – though some may alter brain chemistry. However, some interventions like ECT might alter brain structure, but very grossly or bluntly. Verbal therapies do have the possibility of weakening noxious connections and developing or reinforcing positive ones.

Comparing the Brain to a Computer System

Perhaps the best way to understand this is by comparison with computers. Computer software (e.g., an app) is a set of instructions that tells the computer hardware (electronic components) what to do. But software is separate from the hardware and different from it (software is instructions, bits of information, not electronic components, although they reside in electronic components). Software changes only the electronic state of the hardware's electronic components. In today's computers (though there are ways this can evolve), the software does not alter the nature of the electronic components that comprise the hardware. Different software, data and information cause the hardware to do different things. However, if we took the software out, the hardware would be unchanged.

The brain is different! It's as if we were just hardware (some call the brain 'wetware') and everything that happens changes that hardware. This realization that the structure and chemistry of the brain adapt to literally everything we do or notice or think about or have feelings about is radical! Historically, the mind and the brain have been considered to be separate. Way back, people 'invented' the soul to explain the mind and separate it from the brain. But there is no mind that is separate from the brain. We state that the mind emerges from the brain. The brain and the mind are one! The mind is an operational output of the brain. How we think, feel and behave are manifestations of what our brains do. Disturbed mental health, therefore, could be a signal that we should search for biological abnormalities in the brain or other organs (like we might search for a failed electronic circuit in a computer) that might be responsible. However, if we cannot find objective signs of abnormal organ function in the brain or elsewhere, we should consider implementing non-medical strategies to change mental health because they are properties of our minds. If these less invasive interventions fail, then it is appropriate that clinicians consider pharmaceutical interventions that are known to influence mental state (psychoactive drugs).

We should note that some claim that the mind 'emerges' from the vast complexity of the brain ('emergent' phenomena are considered to be properties of complex systems) and that it is a quantum mechanical effect of the interaction of the billions of nano-level neurons and their trillions of synapses. That is an interesting idea, which unfortunately is above our pay-grade to consider.

Conclusions that Derive from This ─────────────

These realizations can help us understand several things.

For one, we can understand that a lot of mental dysfunction is amenable to self-intervention or to interactions with other people, like therapists or just good friends. In fact, there are few neurologists who doubt that these human-human interactions are therapeutic and also that they alter the structure of the brain and affect how it works.

Another thing we can understand is why pharmaceuticals may not really help and can cause problems because of their side effects. Most importantly, in the case of (non-disease-caused) mental dysfunction, there is no physical disruption or corruption of the brain – though brain chemicals can be changed, so far an unproven hypotheses – that a drug could potentially correct. If there were a true illness behind mental dysfunction, then someone could potentially design an intervention to fix that. Some day scientists may discover that there is an illness, but as of now we are not so enlightened. When there is no disease, most drugs do not correct an illness because there is no illness to correct. This is true even though self-medication with alcohol, marijuana and other substances demonstrates that they influence all normal brains in profound and important ways.

That does not say that pharmaceuticals have no role whatever. If a person is truly "out of it" and a care provider is unable to engage the person despite strenuous efforts, medications can induce mental states that may, at least in certain circumstances, calm a person or otherwise alter the person's state sufficiently so there is an opportunity to intervene verbally. However, drugs can also stupefy the person, engendering a zombie-like state; rather than helping, they can hinder interaction. This may be the best that physicians can do if a person is mentally out of reach, but it isn't often a good starting point for an effective interaction otherwise.

We can even better appreciate the issues here if we awaken to reality. The reality is that it is not clear, in most cases, how even existing psychoactive medications work. Consider an example. When people have moods that oscillate from severe depression to manic excitement (bipolar disorder, formerly called manic-depressive syndrome), doctors prescribe a drug based on Lithium. No one yet knows how Lithium works though there are hypotheses, although some suggest it has a beneficial effect on some people labelled with bipolar disorder.[173] We don't think anyone believes that the bipolar person's brain has a Lithium deficiency (unless there are Lithium batteries in there), but it is doing something chemically to the brain that seems to help. However, no one yet fully understands either what the brain dysfunction is nor what's the effect of the Lithium.

The problem is that many psychoactive drugs are not true treatments of a known biological problem – they don't fix anything, or we are not sure what it is they do 'fix'. They are more akin to analgesics, like Aspirin or acetaminophen, that abate the pain without addressing what is causing the pain. And they can have unpleasant or unhelpful side effects.

173 Lithium: Bipolar disorder and neurodegenerative diseases Possible cellular mechanisms of the therapeutic effects of lithium. F. Marmol. Progress in Neuro-Psychopharmacology & Biological Psychiatry. 32 (2008) 1761–1771. https://pubmed.ncbi.nlm.nih.gov/18789369/. Accessed Mar 23, 2024.

Summary

In summary, here is what we think we know.

Firstly, research seems to be uncovering how the cells of the brain work, connect and interact. Work is underway to create software or mathematical models of at least parts of the brain, but there are many who see this as a hopeless effort. Research also is teaching us that there are brain 'circuits' (chains of neural activation) or what we could call 'collaborations' among different parts of the brain, which occur as we make decisions, emote, speak or hit a piano key.

Secondly, we have come to understand at least the existence of what scientists call 'brain plasticity', the ability of the brain to adapt. This is most clear when a person has an injury that damages a part of the brain. It is possible, over time and with assistance, for a person to relearn lost skills (like speaking and reading) because another part of the brain can take over those functions. This is probably the most obvious case of brain restructuring. However, we believe we know that everything we feel or do or think changes the brain by either forming new connections or making those connections more or less efficient. Brain imaging tells us that.

Thirdly, we know that a great deal of what we call "mental illness" is not an illness, i.e., caused by some sort of insult to the brain (we again refer you to the last Chapter at the end of this Section). Much of the misnamed 'mental illness' should be termed 'mental dysfunction'. Mental dysfunction is amenable to a wide range of therapies that include talking, friendly concern and contact, being loved, seeing concern in another's eyes or just noticing that someone cares. Although it may be necessary in extreme cases to use pharmaceuticals in the case of mental dysfunction, the only true value (at least so far) is to put the person in a state of mind that is open to engaging in those types of interventions. In the case of 'real illness', the appropriate approach is to determine what is wrong biologically and take steps to correct or minimize that using proven therapies, including pharmaceuticals, that help the person recover.

Fourthly, we now realize that whenever someone helps another person, it in some way changes the person's brain and makes it possible for the person to have better approaches to thinking, more effective management of emotions or more adaptive behavior. It is also important to recognize that bad experiences a person has also change the brain. We touch on that further in the chapter on dangerousness.

The mind-brain system represents probably the most mysterious aspect of being human. Humankind that has come to great understandings – the formation of the universe, the role of quantum mechanics in nature and the impact of general relativity on motion – must admit that we may never truly understand the mind and consciousness. There are many theories of consciousness, but the mind looking at itself seems impaired in reaching clear and cogent conclusions as to what it perceives.

What is important here is that we need to recognize that much mental dysfunction is an ordinary reaction to ordinary life, which can be extraordinarily difficult to experience.

Chapter 16: ——— Interview with a Psychiatrist

KEYWORDS: Psychiatrist's Viewpoint, Robbie Campbell, Psychotherapy, Needed Skills, Active Listening, Role of Medication, Recordkeeping, Therapeutic Alliance, Brain Disorders, Eating Disorders Foundation of Canada

ABSTRACT: It should be clear by now that mental health professionals approach mental problems in a variety of ways. In particular, matching someone with a problem with a professional therapist may be a challenge. One of the authors has a friend who is a psychiatrist who offered to reflect on the nature of psychiatry and the elements of medical training that were most pertinent to his professional practice. Dr. Robbie Campbell states that listening is the most important skill in psychiatry; a skill that is valuable and, in fact, essential in many professions, and, indeed, in most relationships. He also notes that medical schools do not teach this most important skill, listening. If it is learned, it is acquired through apprenticeship, when students participate in therapy sessions and observe psychiatrists in action. An important point he makes regards how the burden of recordkeeping, and recording superfluous (though sometimes mandated) information, interferes with the doctor-patient relationship. His assertion that sometimes clinicians use drugs to influence a disturbed person's behavior because the therapist just does not have the time for less invasive interventions, warrants serious consideration by health system designers and administrators. Perhaps the answer is to provide other avenues to therapy or enable care providers to have the time. Dr. Campbell believes (as do many other psychiatrists) that certain problems, for example those labelled as schizophrenia, obsessive-compulsive disorder or bipolar disorder, may reflect biological abnormalities that require long term use of drugs. We did discuss elsewhere that some patients with these labels may eventually graduate from dependence on continuing medication.

Introduction: Get Ready for your Mind to Expand as we Talk to a 'Shrink'! ———

We thought it would be interesting and revealing to ask Dr. Robbie Campbell[174] (see FIGURE 2.16.1), a psychiatrist and friend, to reflect on the nature of his profession. Robbie practices in London, Ontario, Canada and has connections with us through the field of Health Informatics wherein he has an interest in Telepsychiatry – remote therapy supported by video or online linkages.

---

174 https://www.lawsonresearch.ca/scientist/dr-robbie-campbell. Accessed Feb. 10, 2023.

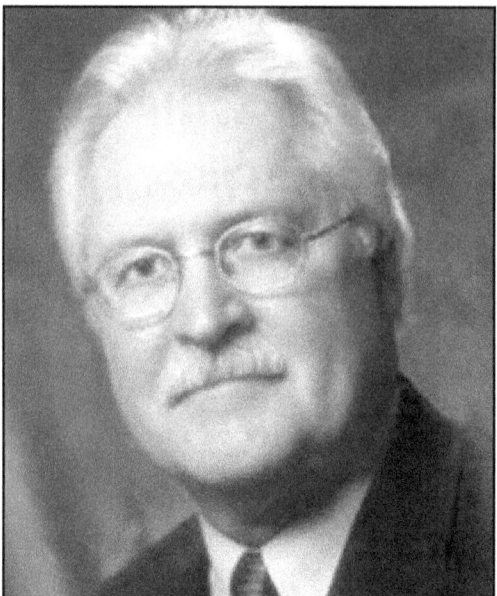

FIGURE 2.16.1: Robbie Campbell, MD, FRCPC

Interviewer: Which skills, acquired before, during or after training, have been of the greatest importance to you as a psychiatrist?

Dr. Campbell: Perhaps the most important skill is listening. Some who enter the field of Psychiatry have a natural ability in that regard, but others seem challenged. Listening is probably a prerequisite to be a good psychiatrist or therapist. It is important to go further than this, however, and to learn to become an effective 'active listener', which I define as "the art of tastefully and constructively interacting in order to form a true therapeutic alliance with the patient." Active listening means that the therapist must deeply engage with the patient and the patient must be convinced the therapist is taking it all in.

———

Interviewer: Are listening skills considered by admissions committees in assessing applicants to psychiatric training programs?

Dr. Campbell: No. During admission deliberations, the primary focus seems to be on applicant's grades and selection committees pay far too much attention to them!

———

Interviewer: Ok. Then, is this skill taught to students during med school or during psychiatric residency programs?

Dr. Campbell: No. It's not taught in med school, and students learn (hopefully) by example from mentors and during other training, such as in supervised individual and group therapy sessions.

This brings up another point. I believe we need more formality in our psychiatric post-medical school programs. Our programs would seem to benefit from an analysis of the competencies we wish to imbue in students and from the definition of the material to which they must be exposed to acquire these competencies.

To do this, we need to do some forward and comprehensive thinking about the roles of psychiatrists and what we expect from them during practice. Listening would be one of these key competencies and there are many others, such as the ability to sense and understand the patient's issues and the approaches to addressing them that will fit with the patient. Right now, programs border on being apprenticeships. However, there are definable areas of knowledge, skills and even attitudes that would better prepare students for the challenges of mental health care. Finally, ensuring that teachers expose students to a wide variety of situations is important so that the students' experience-repertoire is also adequate.

———

Interviewer: What is it that concerns you about today's training programs? What can you say about their graduates? Are they competent in psychotherapy?

Dr. Campbell: We seem to have moved deeply into the digital age, but in a bad way. Today, there tends to be too much emphasis on computer use, data collection, recordkeeping, filling out forms, completing questionnaires, compulsory reporting, etc., in place of fulsome conversation. The therapist seems focused on making sure that nothing is missed record-wise. Unfortunately, the victim of this focus is the doctor-patient relationship or what we will call the therapeutic alliance. The therapist captures the information but the healing inter-action loses out.

In training therapists, we need far greater emphasis on how to listen. The therapeutic value is not just in what patients say, but how they say it. Affect carries very valuable infor-mation and clues to addressing problems. The therapist must grasp the whole and in-depth story and not just focus on the presenting symptoms. This allows seeing and taking into account the forest instead of just the trees.

When the focus is on the immediate symptoms and on prescribing medication, unfortunately, there is often no room left to unravel what is causing the symptoms. There can also be too much emphasis on the now and not enough on what has been the origin of the problems. We need to see how the past, present and future are intimately connected. I guess this is another way of saying we need to acquire a holistic view of the patient's life, especially related to resulting problems.

———

Interviewer: What do you see as the primary uses/value of psychoactive drugs? For what sort of duration?

Dr. Campbell: Psychoactive drugs are very valuable as part of what psychiatrists have to offer but often, because of time and many pres-sures, drugs can become the only thing offered.

It is always better to blend psychotherapy (no matter which of the many flavors) and medica-tion – when necessary – as a package for best results and not focus on either/or. Obviously, different medications are more effective for different presentations and situations. Some drugs are for the short-term and some for the long-term, depending on the presenting symp-toms, history and diagnosis.

The use of drugs is especially important if the patient is highly agitated or unable to engage meaningfully with the therapist. Medication can help create an environment more suitable for interaction and more likely to enable chan-nels of communication with the patient. Think about this like when you have faced a frighten-ing or profoundly upsetting experience, and someone tried to talk to you. You may simply have been out of reach. Medication can make both listening and expression possible for the patient.

———

Interviewer: The literature on state-depen-dent learning seems to indicate that organisms are more likely to forget when they've learned something in one drug state and someone tests their recall in another state. What do you think? Can drugs undermine psychotherapy?

Dr. Campbell: I believe it is important to understand the role of drugs in Psychiatry. One major role is to help the patient achieve a mental and behavioral state that is con-ducive to interacting productively with the psychiatrist. If the patient is terrified, hyper-anxious, morose and deeply depressed, that is a state that is going to frustrate psychotherapy. Psychotherapy is in its essence an intimate and personal conversation intended to uncover and then deal with problems that are besetting the patient. Medication can help calm the patient or sufficiently energize the patient to enhance receptivity and provide that opportunity for a meaningful therapeutic conversation. My experience is that insights and achievements realized by a patient assisted by medication are intact afterwards. In fact, in many cases they are the *sine qua non* (without which, nothing) of patient engagement and resolution.

———

Interviewer: We spoke a bit about record-keeping and how it can negatively impact the encounter with the patient. Can you expand on this?

Dr. Campbell: Recordkeeping is important to remind the therapist of what has been covered, which problems the therapist has or has addressed, and it can serve as a stepping-stone for the next session. It also permits communication with other care providers. The therapist often uses manual computer entry to record the elements of the conversation during the meeting, but this can be very distracting. The focus on recordkeeping can actually be untherapeutic or even anti-therapeutic and make the patient feel unheeded, ignored and unappreciated, thereby detracting from the clinician's goal of a healthy therapeutic relationship. I don't care for the word 'encounter', as it is not a warm description of a meeting and is a rather cold, computeresque term that implies confrontation or a glancing interaction and does not reflect the value of relationship-building in moving towards the resolution of the patient's problems.

———

Interviewer: Are there brain disorders that require long-term medication and what are some examples?

Dr. Campbell: Yes, there are many brain disorders like neurodegenerative diseases, bipolar disorder, schizophrenia and obsessive-compulsive disorder that require long-term

use of medication. The medications target biochemical, structural, genetic and acquired brain factors that would remain problems unless addressed. However, using these drugs demands proper follow-up, monitoring for side effects and scrutinizing their overall efficacy for the patient.

———

Interviewer: Are trainees steeped in the mind-brain dichotomy and related issues? Do they learn about distinguishing matters that may be based on poor thinking, learned bad experiences, etc. versus caused by flawed brain structures/circuits or chemistry? I know that even the formulation of this question is flawed, but I'd like to see what you know/think.

Dr. Campbell: Not in my experience. This may be another area that we should include in a formal Psychiatry curriculum. Clearly, the thing that does the thinking is the brain and it is tightly integrated with the body. This means that pain or a burn can affect the mind and the mind can affect the perception or threat of pain. It may even be best to consider all the nerves in the body together with the brain. Problems with the body, moreover, such as hormone disruptions, can affect the brain and can be at the root of certain psychiatric problems.

———

Interviewer: Do you still find Psychiatry a satisfying profession and what do you most enjoy?

Dr. Campbell: Psychiatry has always been very satisfying and rewarding, as I am in a unique position to help patients understand and resolve their struggles so they can successfully move on and be the best that they can be. I have had a life-long interest in eating disorders and dealing with youth, and continue being a college consulting psychiatrist, as well as

Founder and President of the Eating Disorders Foundation of Canada.[175]

There have been challenges as we move towards working as a team with other professionals and patients. We have a long way to go in defining the role that each team member plays and their interactive responsibilities, especially as the patient must be the most important player on the team. We must also learn how to do a better job at assisting with the transition from the treatment team to the community support team, thereby we can ensure that we do not forget proper follow-up care.

––––––

Interviewer: I would like to personally thank you for both your comments here and for the discussions that led up to them. We have also had some interesting discussions in the past and I wanted you to know how grateful I have always been for them.

175 https://edfc.ca. Accessed Feb. 10,2023.

Chapter 17: ——— Understanding Mind Versus Brain

KEYWORDS: Mind, Brain, Relationship of Brain Dysfunction and Mental Health, Mental Health Problems without Brain Dysfunction, Treatment Versus Intervention.

ABSTRACT: Philosophers have wondered about the relationship between the mind and body for centuries. They and others have pondered if there will ever be lab investigations or brain imaging techniques that will enable us to understand or predict what a person the thinking, feeling or likely to do. Will we ever have biomarkers (biomarkers: abnormal blood test results, genetic findings, images or other physical evidence) of a mental problem? For now, it seems, we have to be content with treating mental problems associated with a diagnosed biological abnormality with medications that we know influence that person's medical problem. When we cannot recognize abnormal biomarkers, it is appropriate to continue to look for them while implementing nonmedicinal interventions. When conventional psychological interventions fail to help a person, it is appropriate to try psychotropic medication in the hope that it will alleviate the problem, even though we have no way of knowing whether the drug is correcting a biological dysfunction or not.

A forewarning: This material may help understand the relationship between the brain and mind. However, it is only an analogy, not a true explanation. We confess to being as or more challenged than others in providing a clear and cogent description of the nature of the mind and its connection with the brain.

Words Have Consequences ———

Words indicate and influence <u>what</u> and <u>how</u> we think about issues. Words, by their very nature, are categorizations; they include certain meanings we wish to connote and exclude others. We use one word and not another to communicate a specific meaning. Related to mental health, we should use 'mental' to refer to the <u>mind</u>, not to the brain.

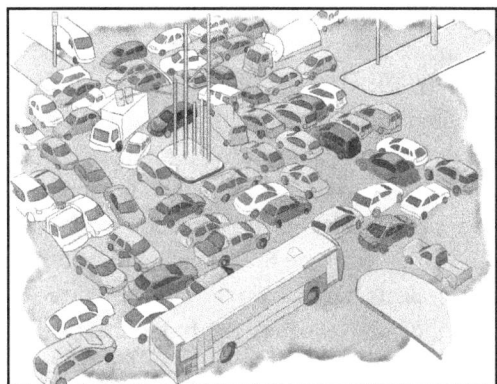

FIGURE 2.17.1: Confusion Leads to Traffic Jams

The Mind and Brain and an Analogy

The mind is an emergent function of the brain. It arises from the brain and appears to have powers proportional to the complexity of the brain. However, the mind is not the brain – the brain is physical – cells, chemicals and connections – the mind is non-physical. To understand that point, consider the following analogy. We use a familiar one traffic and driving.

To present it clearly, we will label our statements with each of the ideas we compare.

TRAFFIC INFRASTRUCTURE: The traffic infrastructure includes the roads, intersections, overpasses, signals, impediments, cars, drivers (or self-driving vehicles) and all the other odds and ends like speed limit signs and speed bumps. We will ask you shortly to consider the traffic infrastructure as the analog of the brain.

TRAFFIC FLOW PATTERN: When cars use a city's roads, a traffic pattern will ensue – a result of how the traffic flows. The cars go up one street, cross intersections, continue ahead, turn and go in a different direction and so on. As the cars participate in this pattern, now and then a traffic jam will occur because of a problem. The problem might be a stalled car, a failed traffic signal, icy roads, sheer volume or any number of other issues. We will also ask you shortly to consider the real time traffic flow pattern being analogous to the functioning of the mind.

THE BRAIN: In the brain, the analogs to the components of the traffic infrastructure are the nerve cells that can be excited and can conduct electrical signals, and the chemicals and circuits that enable the connection of the components of the brain to each other. The brain is like the traffic infrastructure we described above, where the traffic itself is the signals-carrying inter-neuron communication. In fact, we often talk of 'neural traffic'! The electrical or chemical impulses are the analogs of cars.

THE MIND: Now we need to start thinking about the mind. We emphasize that the mind is a non- physical entity. That is the crucial point. We will compare it to a traffic pattern.

TRAFFIC FLOW PATTERN: Consider again a traffic flow pattern and let's add a traffic jam (see FIGURE 2.17.1). Traffic jams too, like the mind, are non-physical. They are descriptions. Both the traffic flow pattern and the traffic jam are results of many cars, many differently thinking drivers with many different destinations and deadlines all sharing the same roads, some of which may be unpassable or in suboptimal condition. Neither the traffic flow pattern nor the jam are themselves objects; we can only perceive the appearance or behavior of the pattern or the result of the jam. To really grasp that non-physicality, take away all the cars and the traffic infrastructure. There is no pattern or jam left over! The traffic infrastructure – cars and roads and everything about them – is physical. However, the patterns and jams are non-physical.

THE BRAIN: The brain is a physical infrastructure (a 'neurological infrastructure') from which the mind emerges.

THE MIND: Yes, the mind is different, very different. It is "I" in each of us and is conscious of itself, but it is analogous to the traffic flow pattern in that it is non-physical. Not sure it's non-physical? Then take away the cells, impulses, chemistry and circuits of the brain: there is no mind left over. It ceases to exist like the traffic flow pattern would ceases to exist without the cars, roads, etc. A difficult matter to grasp in depth, agreed! But the broad idea should be clear.

Pushing the Analogy – Treating the Brain

Now, as we have admitted, all analogies are imperfect – and you might feel that this one is even more so – but let's take it a little further to see if it helps.

TRAFFIC PATTERN: One can consider a traffic jam as 'travel or traffic flow dysfunction'. A traffic jam delays and irritates drivers, potentially making them late for work. It can be a sign of something wrong with the physical traffic infrastructure. If that's the case, civic planners and engineers can physically intervene. They can build more roads, replace intersections with overpasses, use computers to coordinate traffic lights, alter the speed limits… all that is familiar. In other words, they do physical interventions to improve the physical infrastructure and make it more efficient. Unfortunately, as has oft availed, more cars, impatient drivers and just plain impolite behavior can again result in traffic jams, but we will ignore that. Let's assume that our planners and engineers are geniuses and psychosocial Svengalis.

THE BRAIN: If we switch our focus back to the brain, the 'treatment' of the traffic infrastructure is analogous to the treatment of an injured or otherwise physically impaired brain (the neural traffic/neurological infrastructure) using drugs, surgery or other means. Treatment of the brain is a physical treatment of a physical entity that the doctor believes is somehow impaired or inadequate. Doctors act, in effect, as the Neuro-Civil Engineers that address physical brain problems.

Intervening on the Mind – We Can Not <u>Treat</u> the Mind!

We have asserted that the mind arises from the brain's infrastructure and is analogous to the traffic pattern that arises from the traffic infrastructure. An efficient traffic pattern is analogous to a well-functioning mind. However, like what happens in the traffic infrastructure, the mind can become dysfunctional, analogous to a traffic jam happening.

This is the reason we have written this:

Using the term 'mental illness' connotes that we perceive 'mental dysfunction', a problem of the mind, being a 'physical illness', a problem of the brain. In other words, we are effectively claiming that there is something physically or biologically wrong with the brain, sourced in any of the causes of disease – disease etiologies – we have mentioned. However, we have used the traffic analogy to clarify that the mind is a non-physical entity. Surely, we cannot mean that a non-physical entity, the mind, can have something physically wrong with it! You can see the problem and why there is confusion.

In the case of 'illness', which is synonymous (actually, a denotational sememe) with 'physical illness', we judge that the patient's symptoms and signs are real and actually suffered by or existing in the patient. They are exhibitions of something being physically wrong with the person's body. Furthermore, we judge that some pathological agency (like an infectious agent, injury, wear and tear and so on) is causing those symptoms and signs. When we use the term 'mental illness', we inappropriately apply this same meaning to the mind, indicating that we believe there is a similar agency, something physically wrong with the mind. But that cannot be!

Semantics to the Rescue

This is where we realize that the terminological issue is important – sometimes life and death important – making semantics much more than an effete academic matter. It becomes a crucial human issue. This is because a great many of the mental problems we humans face are either:

(1) NOT caused by an anatomical, physiological, physical (collectively: 'organic') agency. In this case, the purported 'treatments' (which usually mean organic corrections or ameliorations of an organic cause) would be pointless.

(2) There is NO cogent evidence of an organic cause that we know about or

(3) There IS an organic cause, but the physician has not searched or searched widely enough to identify it, or the limitations of current science make it impossible to discover

the biologic cause. In these last 2 cases, then any organic treatments are merely symbolic. They only serve as 'place fillers' and merely stand in for a treatment…that 'shot in the dark' we mentioned.

On the Other Hand, There Can be Brain Illness

Some people actually have an illness that causes the brain itself to malfunction. In our analogy above this would be a bad road or a problematic intersection. The brain's malfunction may or may not cause mental dysfunction. So, physical brain malfunction sometimes <u>does</u> cause mental dysfunction. However, there are many people with mental dysfunction despite having a perfectly normal brain. We suppose that it would be possible to say that these latter individuals' minds are sick or ill, but the meaning of 'ill' then is a non-physical ill, a contradiction with what we have said about illness. The term 'mental illness' is effectively an oxymoron – a self-contradiction!

Unless we recognize that 'mental illness' is a problematic phrase, we will green-light inappropriate or even dangerous treatments of highly questionable effectiveness. Inappropriate use of the term mental illness predisposes all of us to look for or to claim there are biologic solutions to mental health problems even when there is no evidence of a such a problem.

On 'Treatment' or 'Intervention'

Just a few words on the term 'treatment', which is also problematic.

It would be far better to always use the broader term, 'intervention'. This is because we associate 'treatment' with organic interventions, such as pharmaceuticals, physical therapy, prosthetics, surgery and the like. There are treatments that may correct for underlying illness of the brain (by altering brain chemistry for example – see https://www.

drugs.com/condition/neurologic-disorder. html (Accessed Feb. 11, 2023)). However, physicians should only use these treatments of known brain illness to treat diagnosed biological abnormalities of the brain. Because of this, most of us associate the term 'treatment' with something that only a professional can do.

Mental interventions, interventions on the mind, are, appropriately, mostly verbal – mood and behavior related. They do not require professional application – patients, relatives, friends and neighbors can intervene to address someone's mental health problems. In the case of mental interventions, physicians sometimes use pharmaceuticals, but they are mainly for the purpose of managing patient symptoms, such as calming the patient or reducing hallucinations or other problems that interfere with interacting with the person. They provide an opportunity for psychotherapy to proceed. **That is, they are <u>not</u> 'treatments' for the mind!**

Sometimes clinicians do use pharmaceuticals to treat what they consider is mental illness – a dysfunction of the brain – e.g., in addressing severe depression of unknown cause, schizophrenic thought disorder or anxiety states. If they do that, clinicians are often using drugs without an understanding of what they are correcting in the brain…and they may not be. In this case, clinicians are acting on beliefs, faith in a drug. They are not acting based on understanding or evidence of biological effects. Maybe this is another example of the art of Medicine! However, if so, it is abstract art! With time, however, if researchers can show that problems of the brain cause problems of the mind that interventions can correct, then that intervention makes medical sense.

Returning to Traffic

To cap this off, perhaps going back to the traffic analog would be worthwhile.

We know we can reduce or eliminate traffic jams by creating more or wider roads, by reducing the number of cars especially at a given time, by eliminating intersections or changing speed limits. These are actual <u>treatments</u> of underlying traffic infrastructure problems and would possibly influence and correct the problems. The roads might have been suboptimal for the purpose of handling traffic, just as some of our brains might not be up to some purposes. Perhaps examples would be a brain injury or a brain affected by some disease.

Intervening on the mind, on the other hand, is like altering the behavior of drivers, such as changing their schedules, preventing rushing and improving driver discipline – interventions on their minds! Indeed, experience has proved that we can influence traffic jams in various ways without changing cars or roads. We can change driver behavior.

Our Minds Can Still Experience 'Jams'!

What is most interesting about this mind-traffic analogy is that history has taught us that, no matter how we address the physical traffic problem (roads, lights, speeds, intersections), there will still be traffic jams! Analogously, no matter how healthy and adequate for normal situations our brains are, situations can push them into a state where coping can fail and we experience the mental equivalent of a traffic Jam, some sort of mental dysfunction! Like roads have limits, so the mind has limits and it may need help!

Now that was challenging! Was it good for you?

VOLUME 2

—————— Section 3 ——————
PUBLIC HEALTH

In the future there may be quite a few quaranteens running around! (based on: https://sites.google.com/view/public-health-edugators/comic-relief/jokes?pli=1).

Last week, I asked my friend if I could pick up any toilet paper at the big-box store. She said, "No. I have a pandemic supply of it!". (Note: easier to understand if you went through it!)

Public Health poster on sale: "Got Polio? Me neither! Thanks, Science!

Many women note that it seems the root of the word 'virus', is 'the Latin word 'vir', which means 'man', so there will never be a cure! Actually, 'virus' is the Latin word for "slimy, liquid, poison"…which seems to substantiate that analysis!

Public Health is a society-level life and death matter. Reflecting on 'death', there was a sign on a fence at the University of Wisconsin in the 1960s that said: "There is no God", (signed) Nietzsche" below which someone had painted: "There is no Nietzsche", (signed) God.

My dad died when we couldn't remember his blood type. As he died, he kept insisting for us to "be positive," but it's hard without him. (https://onelinefun.com/health/).

Preventing childhood obesity. It's as easy as taking candy from a baby! (from: tumblr.tastefullyoffensive.com).

APOLOGIA[176]

When we completed this section, a friend and highly respected Biomedical and Health Informatician, Dr. John H. Holmes[177] at the University of Pennsylvania, kindly read the material and commented on it. John is involved in quantitative Epidemiology in the field of Population Health. He advised that we should address a key matter that has stimulated discussion and debate among Population Health professionals regarding the definition of Public Health. This is a brief interlude to recognize that issue.

To some degree, we have implicitly dealt with some of the issues throughout the books, but by labeling this section 'Public Health' we need to provide some clarification. We write 'implicitly', because we have adhered to the principle that we must consider the entire context of health – what the World Health Organization calls the 'Determinants of Health', not just what the direct care system deals with. We have also emphasized the crucial need for the assessment of the outcomes of any interventions undertaken in the name of treating disease or improving health. Finally, we have written about both the physical and mental (including social) aspects of health, as you see in this volume. We might summarize this by saying we have considered health to be all the aspects of health, and the entire context and nature of the holistic human being.

Historically, what we can call 'Classical' Public Health has focused on – as we have emphasized in this section – the detection of the physical/biomedical threats to health and medical interventions such as vaccination. Reality is that the concept of Public Health must incorporate the logical union of all the issues addressed by 'Classical' Public Health and those addressed by the relatively new field called Population Health. This newer field has not limited itself to what we might call biomedical issues (such as the detection and prevention of diseases), but looks at the much broader picture of the determinants of health such as economics, nutrition, environment, housing, education and all the other influences on a person's health, as well as the impacts of healthcare interventions. It cannot just be that there is an overlap between the two fields; rather there should be a single spanning field that we might call 'Meta-Health'.

We have tried to avoid dancing with the Angels on the head of a pin, that is, "effete distinctions", throughout these books. However, the position of those in Population Health is that we must take a broader perspective in order to truly address the comprehensive health needs of human beings. If you want to read the arguments related to the terms public health and population health, please enjoy these references[178] [179].

Although in the Section on Public Health we emphasize the classical concept of Public Health, we ask that you consider that it was not our intention to limit ourselves or you to that. As you read this material also consider the comments we have included elsewhere on Prevention, Promotion, the critical importance of the assessment of outcomes from any health interventions, as well as our inclusion of both the physical and the mental nature of the human being.

DC

---

176 We use this term to indicate that this is an explanation of the way we have proceeded. It was apparently first used by Justyn Martyr around the year 155, and later used in John Henry Newman's 'Apologia Pro Vita Sua'). It is in no way an apology. https://en.wikipedia.org/wiki/Apologia. Accessed May 23, 2024.

177 https://www.dbei.med.upenn.edu/bio/john-h-holmes-phd-face-facmi. Accessed May 21, 2024.

178 On the Distinction—or Lack of Distinction—Between Population Health and Public Health, Ana V. Diez Roux, Am J Public Health. 2016 April; 106(4): 619–620. https://pubmed.ncbi.nlm.nih.gov/26959262/. Accessed May 21, 2024.

179 Public Health and Population Health: Are They the Same Thing? Dave A. Chokshi, MD, MSc and Namita Seth Mohta, https://www.ncbi.nlm.nih.gov/pmc/articles/PMC7894749/. Accessed May 21, 2024.

Chapter 18: ———— Introduction to Public Health

KEYWORDS: Prevention, Health Maintenance, Humongous Body, Disease Spread, Surveillance, Health Monitoring, Mitigation, Public Health Departments, Models to Detect Cause, Causes of Epidemics, Surge Capacity

ABSTRACT: Individuals and communities are all connected and form a 'humongous body'. The behavior and contributions of each member contributes to the welfare or sickness of others. Public health experts try to relate a person's chances of sickness to their environment. They use information tools to learn if certain physical or social environments are associated with diseases or other problems. Epidemiologists, for example, try to determine if there are air pollutants or other provoking agents in areas with high rates of respiratory disease. In the case of infectious disease outbreaks, Public Health professionals try to find the cause of the infection, to learn how the disease spreads and determine how infectious it is. Public Health experts continuously survey communities or test people, looking for local problems, epidemics or emergent pandemics and seeking the responsible agent. Once the infectious agent is determined, they promote measures for mitigating spread and provide or foster the development of vaccines and therapeutics to counter the infections.

Introduction —————

Today's medical and surgical treatments are almost miraculous! Newspapers celebrate medical miracles almost daily. Surely, they should be the primary focus of our investments in health care! Or should they?

We need to answer this question intelligently and, to do that, we need to realize that there is another crucial component of the healthcare system: Public Health. To really appreciate Public Health and its value, recognize that we have done nothing in health care that has been of greater value than what Public Health has delivered. Not even close! True, we have developed what seem like miracle drugs. Sure, we can test for and diagnose a zillion problems. Yes, we can now replace a person's heart or lungs. Yep, we have evolved psychosocial methods of helping people through the mental challenges that beset their lives. We have done many great things. However, none of these approximate the life-improvement and lifesaving achieved through Public Health. Relatively low-tech solutions like sanitization (including flush toilets and fresh water) and immunization have produced marvellous, but often unappreciated, health benefits.

To help appreciate this, we will share the story of Dr. Methuselah, DPH (Doctor of Public Health) with you. We hope you enjoy it.

THE STORY OF DR. METHUSELAH DPH

Let us start by admitting that Dr. Methuselah's birth-date is a mystery; it could be off by a thousand or more years. Even stranger, Dr. Methuselah's gender is uncertain, as well as the spelling of the good doctor's name. So, let's use 'Dr. M' as we examine a life well lived. We will start our story from when Dr. M was relatively young and medical science itself was in its infancy.

The first reporting about Dr. M was before the year 1000 during travels in Arabia and China, when smallpox (now known to be caused by a virus) wreaked havoc. The Chinese documented that journey because they recognized the importance of an insight Dr. M had about smallpox: noticing that people who previously had smallpox did not get it again. That seems simple but it had powerful implications.

It took a while for those implications to become obvious, though. Between then and the 1600s, while travelling around the world Dr. M promoted the idea of 'pre-infecting' a person. The idea was to give a person a less threatening infection of smallpox than the usual. In other words, Dr. M suggested introducing a person to smallpox artificially. We now call this 'inoculation' or 'vaccination' but at the time, it was known as 'vari-olation'. Back then, however, it was a bit gory: infective material from the pustules of a person with smallpox was placed on the skin of a healthy person and punctures were made so that a bit of the infectious material entered the body. If everything went well, the person got a relatively mild smallpox infection, rather than the full-blown variety they would get naturally. Still, some people died, but only about 1% compared to over 30% (for kids 80%) who died from the natural infection. If we realize that possibly billions of people have been infected over human history and that up to 500 million (!) died even during the 1900s because they were not vaccinated, this was a very meaningful impact! Later, during the 1700s, better techniques were developed, especially the use of cowpox as the artificial infectious agent, dramatically further reducing mortality. So began the public revelation of the life-saving legacy of Dr. M!

We'll skip a few decades and pick up Dr. M's escapades over a hundred years later. Now a bit older, but still comparatively young, we learn of another success. Dr. M turned up in Britain in London late in the 1800s. A horrible disease called cholera was then killing tens of thousands of people in Britain and millions around the world but no one knew what caused it. Scientists had not yet discovered bacteria (which turned out to be the cause), let alone the far tinier viruses. Many, then, believed that disease was caused by something called 'miasma', a word for unpleasant odors like those from decayed flesh or the bodies of sick people. They even wore 'nosegays' to ward off stinks with more pleasant scents (the medical mask of the day?). In London, Dr. M did some detective work and discovered that a source of drinking water was the problem. Sewage was contaminating it and causing cholera. Dr. M's simple solution was the separation of drinking water from sewage. That simple intervention saved uncounted lives!

By the 1900s, Dr. Methuselah was sort of young-to-middle aged, but still very active, thoughtful and effective. People began to listen carefully to the doctor because they saw valuable effects. One of these effects was around 1918 when Dr. M arrived in the United States during the Spanish Flu epidemic. This hit as the First World War was ending and the disbanding of armies sent people back to their homelands, often carrying the illness to others. Here Dr. M saw the value of physical separation among infected people as a way of reducing transmission from one person to another, even though the cause of the Flu was a mystery. Unfortunately, Dr. M was getting a bit older and was not as carefully listened to. Despite this, Dr. M's effects probably saved millions, albeit that millions succumbed to the influenza.

All along the way, Dr. M was having powerful effects. Another of these was the mitigation of the polio epidemic in the 1940s and 1950s in the United States. Dr. M demonstrated that a virus caused polio and Dr. M. stimulated the production of a vaccine to prevent the disease. The good news was that we had come a long way since Arabia, so the vaccine was safe! When millions of people were vaccinated (by injection or an oral agent) millions of infections were prevented. However, at one time, thousands of children were in horrible contraptions called 'iron lungs' (there were some wooden ones in Canada) that helped them to breathe when the virus was active in their bodies damaging their nerves. Even today we see the aftereffects of that epidemic. Those who were infected and survived have what we call 'post-polio syndrome', significant muscle weakness that affects their ability to function.

Unfortunately, age bias was catching up with Dr. M, who was still very active and functional but sort of type-cast like so many of our older people who are sidelined *because of gray hair and a few wrinkles. People began to forget what Dr. M had done and the massive impacts that resulted! The truth was that society began ignoring Dr. M. New miracle drugs and dramatic surgeries captured their attention and they forgot the great doctor.*

It even got worse! In the latter part of the 1900s and early 2000's, there seemed to emerge an almost systematic attempt to pretend that Dr. M was no longer functional, definitely no longer relevant and surely no longer effective. A kind of 'revisionism' kicked in and some seemed to deny Dr. M's work, ignoring or curtailing the establishment of disease testing facilities, reporting systems and vaccine development labs. The funding that had enabled Dr. M's work dried up. Over the course of time, quite a following of Dr. M had emerged – people who called themselves 'Public Health professionals'. However, they were also sidelined, declared redundant and their funding reduced or cancelled. Political leaders ripped out many of the agencies Dr. M. had spawned. It seemed that Dr. M was destined for the dustbin of history. How easily we forget!

Then something terrible happened: A virus called SARS-CoV-2 that caused the disease COVID-19 appeared. The likelihood of infectious agents like it arising was predictable and actually predicted. There had been recent outbreaks of Ebola, SARS, MERS, ZIKA and a host of other viral illnesses. But the predictions were ignored; early alarms were suppressed. National agencies did almost nothing to get ready for what was likely inevitable.

COVID-19 suddenly reawakened the world to the importance of Dr. M.! People belatedly realized that Public Health care underpins trillions of dollars of the domestic products of every nation on the planet. Suddenly the price was clear and Dr. M's value became obvious even to those whose heads were in the sand ignoring history.

As it turned out, ignoring Dr. M cost the world millions of lives, trillions of dollars of waste and years of delayed progress. Dr. M now shines for all to see and has been called back to active duty! Or so we hope! Long live Dr. M!

The moral of this story is that we must understand which aspect of health care has had the greatest overall effect on all of humankind. That is Public Health! Then we must put our money behind rebuilding our Public Health system.

What is Public Health?

The easiest way to understand the nature of Public Health is to conceive of a 'Humongous Body' (a body of bodies) comprising all of us with human bodies who make up the population of a community, a state or province, a country or the entire Earth. We have expanded on that in the Appendix related to misinformation and disinformation. Public Health is to the Humongous Body what health care is to the individual. The human body is a complex system of cells and organs, while the Humongous Body is a complex system of people. Furthermore, much as the human body can get sick, the Humongous Body can get sick. Physicians try to keep each person from getting sick; Public Health tries to keep one sick person from getting everyone sick and helping those who do.

ON 'HUMONGOUS BODY'

We truly wish we had another term in English to express an entire population, for example of a country, in a better way. But we do not seem to have a word. The alternatives are words like 'the public', 'the people' – as in "We the people…" – 'the population', 'the populace', 'society' and the like. However, we did not like any of these. The 'Humongous Body' phrase also allowed us to draw the connection of 'humon-gous' to 'hum-anity'. German has the term: 'Volk', which embodies the idea but doesn't work when translated as 'folk' in English. We hope we are forgiven or at least excused for this one!

It is obviously true that we cannot get that Humongous Body into an office to directly examine and treat it. So, the Public Health system creates a virtual office that views and assesses the Humongous Body through physicians' and other care providers' reports and the results of testing (physicians must report some test results to the Public Health system) regarding individual human bodies. The Public Health system does this to determine if anything is wrong and then publishes the health status of the Humongous Body so that everybody knows.

If the Public Health "office" detects a problem and diagnoses a cause, then, much like an individual doctor does, it treats that problem. The treatments (or, better, 'interventions') used are different from those in the physician's office, but they are treatments, nonetheless. They include interventions such as keeping sick individuals separate (isolated, quarantined) so that others don't get sick, and monitoring to ensure personnel care for those isolated and return them to productive life. The Public Health "office" also tries to prevent illness through the development and application of vaccinations and other medical intermediations.

The Public Health "office" is also particularly aware of environments. It recognizes that everything around individuals influences the Humongous Body. Air pollution, contaminated water, even areas where people can't get nutritious food (those 'food deserts') all contribute to the well being of the Humongous Body and the individuals that comprise it. We call these the 'determinants of health'.

Much like a physician in the medical office, Public Health observes, diagnoses, treats, follows up to make sure all went well and institutes preventive measures.

What would happen if the physician in the medical office didn't listen or observe the patient? I think we all know that diagnosis would not be possible. The same is true of the Public Health system. However, because the Humongous Body is spread all over the surface of planet Earth, we must do observation remotely through distributed 'sensors' (such as individual physicians, other care providers and labs). What's more, this observation must be continuous and what we find we must widely share. If something happens to a part of the Humongous Body in Mongolia, people in Peru need to know about it. With many of the illnesses addressed by Public Health (really, any illness that affects bunches of people, especially communicable ones), whatever happens elsewhere is a model of what can and will happen anywhere. The inhabitants of this planet are so physically connected through the exchange of food and via personal transportation and shared air that illnesses spread everywhere they possibly can. Among the worst threats in this regard are viruses, but other diseases can do the same, albeit possibly less rapidly.

Upon detecting a problem, the Public Health system must be able to communicate the problem widely and to intervene, or the inevitable will happen and everyone, possibly billions, will suffer. We've mentioned some of the interventions, but perhaps the most important one is communication, so that everyone is aware of the threat. One can think of the Public Health system as a security system that alarms about an intruder but also calls the cops! When it comes to the matters addressed by Public Health, no news is not good news; it is very bad news. The smoke alarm can't be inoperative when the 'house' is on fire or lives may be in danger!

A FEW DEFINITIONS

There are several terms used in Public Health are worthy of a clear definition here:

- **Epidemic:** *a disease (usually infectious – communicable – but sometimes applied to other medical problems, such as obesity or ingestible toxins) that is widespread, especially one that is rapidly spread within a single country. It comes from the Greek prefix 'epi', which means 'on' and the Greek word 'demos', which means 'people'. In Principles of Epidemiology*, 15 cases per 100,000 is the numeric threshold for declaring an epidemic. Epidemiology is the scientific study of epidemics and other matters the impact populations.*
- **Pandemic:** *an epidemic that has affected multiple countries or the whole world ('pan' means 'all'). There is ambiguity in the distinction between epidemics and pandemics.*
- **R-Factor (R0):** *reproduction factor; an indicator expressing the probability that an infected person will pass the disease to a number*

of others. R0=4 means that, on average, one infected person will communicate the disease to 4 others.

- **Mathematical Modeling:** *systems of equations that use historical and new data and current assumptions (about the rate of spread, the effects of mitigation, and many other factors) to provide projections about the likely status of a population enduring the effects of an infectious disease.*

Phases of epidemic intervention:

- **Surveillance:** *monitoring populations to detect an outbreak of disease.*
- **Containment:** *having detected a disease outbreak, containment involves contacting infected individuals and discovering how they got the disease and whom they might have contacted and thereby infected. This is the attempt to control disease spread.*
- **Mitigation:** *steps to control the spread of a disease that has escaped containment, i.e., despite locating all contacts, others have been infected. The disease is effectively out of control. To limit the rate of disease spread, it becomes necessary to test those who present with symptoms, but this is done in the face of the realization that others are infected and will present later. Healthcare personnel must wear personal protective equipment (PPE) that reduces the likelihood of their becoming infected. The populations must also undertake efforts to reduce spread (hand washing, avoiding crowds or certain food, for example.) The means of spread determines the type of PPE. A respiratory virus spread by airborne droplets or aerosols will require care providers to wear masks relatively impervious to microscopic droplets, while an intestinal virus might require care in handling or avoiding bodily wastes.*
- **Post Containment Surveillance:** *once contained or if the disease circulates in the population long-term, surveillance and containment become crucial again.*

* *Principles of Epidemiology, Third Edition). Atlanta, Georgia: Centers for Disease Control and Prevention. 2012..*

The Capabilities Public Health Needs ───────────

A doctor's office has a variety of tools that help in observing the patient, such as stethoscopes and otoscopes. Furthermore, the doctor can send someone for testing to a laboratory or imaging center. The primary tool of Public Health is surveillance and the laboratory. However, the lab must receive things (saliva, blood, urine, tissue, sewage) to test, so the Public Health system has sensors in the community: medical agencies. These agencies enable Public Health practitioners (but not necessarily all medical doctors) to learn which illness are extant, where illnesses are likely to occur, and the characteristics of the people and communities most likely to become afflicted.

Some medical practices even serve as 'Sentinel Practices' that maintain a special relationship with Public Health and serve as early warning sensors. All physicians must report some diagnoses, like sexually transmitted diseases (STDs), to the Public Health authorities. In addition, we must expand the range of reportable illnesses during an epidemic. Of course, there must be another mechanism, the research and development facilities that create the treatments or preventive measures, as well as medical, administrative and technical staff distributed across all of these. As will become clear shortly, there is even more that we must add to this to properly deal with emergencies. Maybe we should conceptualize the Public Health system more as a variegated, distributed, world-wide virtual hospital that sits over and blends into the existing healthcare system.

In the case of the usual doctor's office or hospital, treatments are often available in the pharmacy down the street. Of course, sometimes they are new and might be out of stock but usually it won't be long until they are available. In Public Health, we create many of the interventions and treatments only after we detect the illness, so the Public Health 'pharmacy' needs to be more like a machine or a factory. This mechanism must be able to create the treatment in real time and then produce it in vast quantities to at least contain the illness, if not eliminate it.

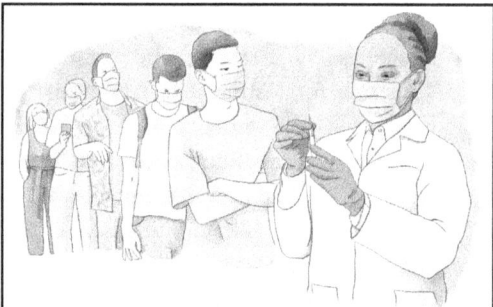

FIGURE 2.18.1: Dr. M. Vaccinating

The Requirements for Realizing Dr. M's Legacy (FIGURE 2.18.1) ⎯⎯

Actually consummating Dr. M's legacy generates a number of significant challenges:

1. We must have a means of continuously monitoring the health of the human beings across the planet. This means that there must be a connection to every locus of clinical practice, offices, hospitals, care facilities for the elderly, laboratories, mobile care providers, and the to Internet so anyone can access it.

2. There must be a mechanism for noticing and diagnosing disturbances to that health and there must be requirements for and ways of communicating that information to central authorities, who must have accommodations for their work.

3. We must have a wide-reaching way of communicating with the public to make them aware of the danger, to educate them on how to avoid infection and what to do if they are concerned they are infected.

4. We must have the resources (people, training, equipment, supplies, facilities, funding) for creating interventions (like therapeutics and vaccines) that will prevent, contain or eliminate threats to the health of the public.

5. We must have facilities for housing and caring for the sick and recovering, including isolation in their own abodes.

6. We must have a means of ensuring that we undertake the intervention process efficiently, and carry it out to completion. We must also ensure that the threat does not recur, which goes back to the continuous monitoring.

The 'Providers' of Public Health ⎯

In these books, we have mentioned a wide array of healthcare workers who assist in the day-to-day healthcare system. We augment these people with specialists in the Public Health system, such as specially trained doctors and allied care providers, researchers, administrators and support staff of many kinds. They must have formal training in Public Health to take the types of roles we have cited.

Beyond these day-to-day staff, outbreaks of illness require both the virtually complete engagement of the existing health system staff, as well as many other staff to handle the overload that an outbreak creates. What's more, there may need to be reserve facilities available for when the volume of required care goes beyond what the existing system can handle. This means that public health virtually demands a 'reserve army' of healthcare people we can call to service in an emergency. The military finds this necessary and it is equally if not more important related to Public Health. It is worth noting that the federal Public Health Service in the United States is a uniformed paramilitary service.

Thoughts About Innovation Related to Public Health ⎯⎯⎯

The authors are not Public Health practitioners. However, we have spent many years teaching and promoting the concepts of Public Health, including surveillance based on community accessible data, and the need for an adequate, functional and effective Public Health system. People seem to largely forget or ignore past public health efforts and their contributions. However, the COVID-19 pandemic emergency provided a real and present stimulus to think about worthwhile suggestions that would make a difference in the next pandemic, which is as inevitable as this one was. Perhaps ears are more prepared to hear these ideas now that the sound of the populace's crying and grumbling is so loud, and the reality of the fiscal implications are so clear. While we do not pretend that these suggestions are the only ones, the best ones or are fully adequate, we do believe that they would make a difference.

Our future and effective Public Health system must have the following capabilities:

1. **Researchers can implement realistic models to reduce person-to-person spread of infection.**

2. **Independent, multiple-use and dedicated-to-epidemics care facilities, with high-volume negative pressure air circulation, electrostatic or ultraviolet air decontamination and secure isolation fitted with modern information and communications technology.** This would dramatically reduce the possibility of infecting others, particularly the healthcare workers so crucial to patient recovery.

3. **Spare capacity, fully automated, adaptable, laboratory testing facilities, including reagent production, augmented by high volume, distributable testing apparatus.** The COVID-19 epidemic showed that testing is crucial and that it is extremely difficult to ramp up. Furthermore, centralized testing has inherent limitations at least associated with specimen transport. Delays in diagnosing infection inevitably results in uncontrollable spread.

4. **Vaccine and therapeutics research and production facilities.** This refers to the development of research and rapid production capabilities to produce 100s of millions of units of vaccines, therapeutic or other required agents.

5. **Stockpiled oxygen, oxygen production facilities and/or oxygen concentrators.**

6. **Locally stockpiled, basic Personal Protective Equipment** (PPE: N95 and hooded masks, surgical masks, gowns, gloves) plus localized extreme PPE (full hazmat suits with filtered air circulation). The lack of adequate PPE during the COVID-19 pandemic doomed many care workers to infection and some to death.

7. **Access to world-wide and country-level Public Health information systems** (including continuous health monitoring data, predictive modelling capabilities and reporting). Based on the need for continuous and widespread monitoring, a Public Health information system is mission critical. Ideally, it would have digital connectivity to existing hospital and practice information systems.

8. **A pre-existing telehealth communications system.** The need for communications and transparency during epidemics is fundamental, both to receive and output every kind of information, including public education material. In the face of a pandemic, the isolation of the population demands the existence of ubiquitous Internet connectivity and availability of workstations, if the economy is to be able to function.

9. **Online pandemic plans and a ready governmental infrastructure backed up with training and regular drills.** Often, we develop plans and then lose

them in a file cabinet somewhere. This happened in COVID-19, and we can avoid that by having plans easily and widely available online. Periodic 'epidemic games' (similar to war games) based on the plan and regular updating are also crucial.

10. **Simple ventilators or CPAP machines.** Many of the viral plagues affect our pulmonary system and a variety of forms of artificial oxygenation are essential. Often today's equipment is overly complicated and based on electronics that is not robust on the shelf. There are answers to this (see Geiger counter anecdote below).

11. **Stockpiled suites of basic clinical monitoring equipment:** oximeters, HR and BP monitors, and imaging technology. As we did during COVID with ventilators and PPE, we must stockpile basic monitoring equipment in large numbers. Equipment like this could likely be periodically subject to sale and replacement to ensure viability.

12. **A reserve Public Health staff 'army' with a command-and-control system.** Intensive care of patients requires properly trained and experienced professionals. Much as in the military, a reserve of people is necessary. We must prepare and register healthcare workers for call-up during emergencies. Leadership of called-up personnel is crucial. Though few who dedicate their lives to health care would ever expect such, there must be a method of recognizing heroism during epidemics. The danger endured is akin to what soldiers face in battle and the awarding of special recognition both posthumously and to survivors is both fitting and essential. A Medal of Honor, bronze and silver stars, as well as purple hearts are all in the range of an appropriate responses.

THE GEIGER COUNTER FOR THE POST-NUCLEAR HOLOCAUST

When DC was a Physics student in high school in the United States in the 1960s, several students found stored material in the school basement that had been placed there by the Civil Defense organization. It was for use in the event of a nuclear war. Our class "borrowed" a Geiger counter (a device used to detect and measure nuclear radiation) from this collection. We learned a great deal using the device and, luckily, it was not needed for its intended purpose. Many years later, DC purchased an identical unit on eBay, as thousands were declared redundant. The devices had been manufactured in the late 1940s or early 1950s and are fully functional over 70 years later. The unit is easily disassembled and the secret to its longevity is clear. It is very simple, uses large discrete components (resistors and capacitors – not fancy integrated circuits that are prone to failure), is very mechanically robust and its batteries are placed in such a way that their degradation will not damage the electronic circuitry. Equipment like this should be a model for other emergency apparatus. There is nothing standing in the way of creating a basic ventilator (a breathing-support machine), especially when one considers that the fall back in the absence of one is a person hand-squeezing a rubber bag to force air into the patient's lungs. We may need highly sophisticated equipment in day-to-day Medicine, but emergencies require what some have called 'meatball Medicine', functional and effective but simple and robust devices and protocols that remain operable long-term.

Community Capacity in Normal Times and During Epidemics ———

People are frightened when they learn about infectious diseases, especially new ones, threatening their health. How frightened and terrified they become relates to the number of people seriously harmed by the disorder, its rate of transmission, the publicity given the disorder, how it behaves and what interventions are available to prevent and mitigate harm. What they are unaware of is that this capacity issue is prevalent.

In America, fear increased when people realized that Public Health capacity was insufficient to test everyone for the COVID-19 virus, and that America might not have the resources, including ventilators and antiviral drugs, necessary to treat the large number of victims.

To reduce harm and allay fears, communities must have the surge capacity allowing them to isolate and treat infected people. They also must have the human resources and testing facilities necessary to learn, as soon as possible, who is infected and consequently communicable, and the characteristics of people the disease is most likely to infect. People with known infections, whether symptomatic or not, can isolate themselves to prevent infecting others.

Most citizens don't know about health system performance during pandemics or in more normal times. This information is not available as governments don't adequately measure performance or inform the public about how many people realize benefit or harm from health system activities. However, there are some aspects of the health system performance that are highly visible if we look. We can see some evidence of the day-to-day performance of health systems, its resilience in the face of epidemics.

One simple indicator of health system resilience – or the lack thereof – is the response of emergency departments and other care facilities to the increased community needs in winter when heart problems increase because sedentary people exert themselves shoveling snow. Some provinces belatedly issue advisories and reduce elective (pre-planned) admissions because the hospitals have exceeded capacity even though the annual surge in shoveling-related admissions is predictable. Others complain loudly that capacity becomes insufficient when staff take either summer holidays or winter vacations. These are well-documented examples where people suffer because of the lack of health services capacity and, again, they are predictable, and administrators could avoid the inevitable crunch by planning ahead.

Another indicator of overburdened health system capacity is premature discharge from Intensive Care Units. This indicator is normally invisible to the public. However, physicians who work in a hospital will have experienced how often administrators insist on premature ICU discharge because of insufficient capacity.

Unfortunately, in Canada and also in some parts of the USA, clinicians have been complicit in efforts by health services administrators and Provincial governments to reduce cost even if it means reducing access. Doctors and nurses have not screamed when forced to provide less than optimal care because of resource shortages or misallocated resources.

Community engagement might encourage regulators, clinicians, and health services administrators to create appropriate resources for normal times and for whenever there are surges in demand, like what happens in a pandemic.

Chapter 19: —————— The Pandemic as Lens

KEYWORDS: Healthcare Implications of Pandemic, Viruses, R-naught, R_0, Information Sharing, Effects of Social Determinants, Policy. Pandemic as Model, Testing Problems, Treatment, Vaccination, Convalescent Sera, Therapeutics, Corona Viruses, Masking, Distancing, Impacts on Education, U.S. Deaths, Global Deaths, Healthcare Workers' Heroism

ABSTRACT: The COVID-19 pandemic and communities' response to it is instructive of the tools and methods physicians in general, as well as epidemiologists and public health experts, use to learn about the determinants of overall health and the agents that cause disease. COVID showed that agencies could collaborate to develop immunizations to prevent transmission of life-threatening illness. It demonstrated that agencies could use modern information tools to identify behaviors that could help people avoid illness. They could also learn who might become ill, seriously ill or even threatened with death, and to intervene to help or care for them. Success required that various elements of the health care system – including primary care professionals, hospitals and communities – collaborate, share information and implement preventive interventions or remedies for those who fall ill. Despite a degree of success, the pandemic revealed that the components of the healthcare system suffer from lack of integration, lack of information, poor communication and a degree of inertia in responding to a major healthcare crisis. These limitations exist at every level and negatively affect the quality of care despite enormous investment in the system and the heroic efforts of individual health professionals.

Introduction

Death, societal disruption, overflowing hospitals, financial dislocation – usually we read about these in sci fi novels when some predatory aliens have come to Earth to destroy or enslave humanity or to hijack its resources. We only wish that what we imagine were science fiction!

In 2020, the entire planet faced off against an alien-like invader. However, it was not a life form from another star system, and some even question if it is truly a form of life. This invader was a virus.

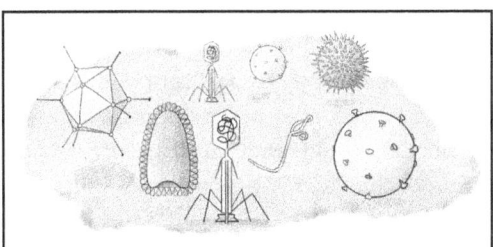

FIGURE 2.19.1: There Are Many Types of Viruses

Either secondary to your own experience or through reading about COVID-19, you are likely familiar with what happened and what continues to happen as COVID, like other viruses, evolves. FIGURE 2.19.1 illustrates that there are many types of viruses

The skinny on a very complicated and wide-ranging event is that a virus, normally resident in animals, mutated, enabling it to infect people.[180] Through the wonders of air travel, infected but unaware (asymptomatic, pre-symptomatic or minimally symptomatic) people, serving as unsuspecting 'mules' like those used by drug smugglers, brought the virus to almost every country on the planet. Those travelers, in turn, infected unwary residents, who then shared it with some of the people they encountered. Each infected person seemed to transmit the virus on average to 2 or 3 other people. (R_0 – 'R-naught' – between 2 and 2.5).[181] [182] Although COVID-19, at least thus far, is less infective than measles (measles R_0 = 12-18), the spread of infections is exponential, affecting an ever-increasing number of people. R_0, the transmissibility rate, is different for different viruses and populations. Mitigation (masks, handwashing, social distancing) efforts reduce R_0, which means that the number of people an infected person infects is dependent on preventive actions, the environment and the population as well as the infective agent.

Very quickly, the virus brought virtually the entire world's population to its knees, interfered with education, and made many people sick or dead. The good news is that reducing the R_0 below 1 – so that it takes more than one infected person to pass on the disease to another person, gradually reduces the number of infections – and results in the eventual eradication of the virus. Wearing masks and social distancing are immediately available ways achieve this. However, we also need to realize that viruses that kill all their victims cannot propagate because the virus dies too! Lucky for the viruses, they generally mutate, which can result in their becoming less deadly, but, if we think about that we can see that transmission is likely!

A favorite sport during and after the pandemic has been attempting to indict different agents or agencies for originating or spreading the contagion or failing to respond quickly enough to halt its spread and to properly treat its victims. We propose to use the pandemic for a more productive purpose: illustrating what our books are all about.

Our Healthcare "System" ————

> **Viruses are one of the many causes of human disease and disability**

The reader is likely aware that viruses are just one of the causes of disease. We have elucidated many other causes – etiologies. We have also elected to detail some because they are common or illustrate key ideas. Remember, the primary purposes of health care are to improve or maintain comfort, function and life expectancy by preventing, detecting and identifying (diagnosing), treating, curing or mitigating diseases or their impacts. Here we will use COVID-19 as an example of a common form of disease – a virus. Luckily, most viruses are not as devastating as this one was.

> **The primary purposes of the healthcare system are to address illness and other health problems and help people maintain their health**

The healthcare system, really a constellation of systems, embodies the people, mechanisms and facilities to address illness and maintain

---

180 https://nationalinterest.org/blog/buzz/how-do-new-viruses-emerge-144127. Accessed Aug 13, 2023.
181 https://www.nytimes.com/2020/04/23/world/europe/coronavirus-R0-explainer.html. Accessed Aug 13, 2023.
182 R_0 indicates how many people on average a person with the virus infects. For comparison, rubella has an R_0 = 6-7 and mumps' R_0 = 4-7.

health. COVID-19 exposed this set of systems as being at best loosely integrated, and therefore often an obstacle to effectively limiting the pandemic. For example, many hospitals amalgamate into groups, but these groups do not coordinate or work with other hospitals and agencies. This frustrated much-needed inter-institutional resources sharing during the pandemic.

An even greater problem is that we seldom design and implement the components of our healthcare system to collaborate related to information capture, analysis and sharing. We should share information to learn if an increase in the problems experienced in a medical setting is a one-off or is a sign of a more systemic issue, for example an impending pandemic. We should also share information so we can determine which interventions help, harm or just waste resources. However, physicians' offices or clinics, hospitals, testing facilities, agencies involved in health prevention and promotion, Public Health organizations, the mental health system and so on largely operate as independent entities that don't share information. COVID-19 revealed this a significant problem with mortal consequences.

> **The healthcare system comprises many components intended to work together to deal with healthcare problems**

Information for Care

We have made much ado in our books about clinical records, the need for information, and the challenges of capturing, sharing and analyzing health information. Records are crucial to support care and to ensure care is effective. Imagine what would happen in a business if Marketing, Sales, Manufacturing, Maintenance and Finance did not share information. Think of all the problems Marketing could cause if it purchased millions of dollars of advertising for a discontinued or dangerous product, or

Finance did not share information about cuts to the advertising budget. Information is the organization's basis for decision-making and productive action. It is the lifeblood of an organization. Not sharing information would be like cutting off the blood supply to a body part – rendering it dysfunctional or dead. Capturing, analyzing and sharing information during the pandemic caused significant healthcare organizational and Public Health care problems, some of which we will mention. Not at all surprising if you remember the adage: "you can't manage what you don't measure".

> **Information is the lifeblood of the healthcare system and essential for patient care**

The Societal Environment of Health Care

The societal health environment, which the World Health Organization has called the 'social determinants of health', was another key aspect of health care in the pandemic. Where and how people live, what they eat, their age, their existing health and their economic state, all affect health and the potential impacts of disease. The pandemic has brought this out ever so clearly. We have become aware that color of skin, poverty, crowding, age and lack of access to many services resulted in disproportionately serious illness and death. This has made it obvious that environments condition health and health care and that neither health nor health care is distributed equitably to all people.

During the pandemic, people infected by COVID-19 were capable of transmitting the virus to anyone they contacted, and the virus did not distinguish between rich and poor. However, less well-off people found it more difficult to escape from crowding and, being less healthy and less-well cared for, were more vulnerable to infection and more likely to suffer more dire consequences. This describes the situation well: *"Researchers from University of Illinois at Urbana-Champaign and DePaul University analyzed data from seven US agencies and organizations ... They found that a 1.0% increase in a county's income inequality was associated with a 2.0% increase in COVID-19 infection and a 3.0% rise in related deaths".*[183]

Furthermore, in long term care organizations, staff, many of whom need several jobs to support themselves and their families, served as vectors for the virus, bringing infection and death to residents who were otherwise isolated.

> **The characteristics of society affect the health of people and the potential of the healthcare system to help people**

Funding and Policy ————————

In these books, we have underscored the necessity of coordination, proper funding, the need to determine if our healthcare investments are truly productive. However, we perhaps have not really paid adequate attention to the devastating outcomes of the failure of leadership. These leadership issues include reasonable prognostication regarding threats, the planning and proper placement and allocation of healthcare resources, the availability of care, the accessibility of needed resources and the maintenance of community health by governments and those agencies directly responsible for health care. One of the problems is that many healthcare administrators are operating in the dark.[184] They lack information systems that would enable them to learn in real time about the health status of communities and the effectiveness of interventions. In many ways

the system behaves as a hearing- and vision-impaired person unaided by compensatory skills and tools.

We also needed leadership from the care providers, such as physicians and allied providers, ensuring that what they did was effective and not harmful.

Then there is our personal leadership of our own care. In the case of COVID-19, this involved recognizing the personal responsibility for minimizing the possibility of becoming infected and thereby endangering healthcare providers and others. This required becoming aware of the nature of infectious contagion, physical distancing, hand washing, avoiding crowds and wearing a mask.

COVID-19 brought into bas relief the crucial importance of leadership at every level. International agencies like the WHO, Presidents and Prime Ministers, healthcare agencies like the CDC and FDA, governors, premiers, mayors and agency administrators all, at the very best, fell short and, with very few exceptions, improperly and inadequately dealt with the pandemic, operating from a state of morbid denial or political bias. Worse, some failed miserably, and many died as a result.

> **The coordination and integration of healthcare agencies and what they do depends on excellent and intelligent leadership**

One of the most perverse phenomena during the pandemic was the politicisation of the disease and of the interventions that might help victims. Dictators and demagogues and even some Free World leaders used the pandemic to amplify their ideologies and promote their chauvinism.

183 https://www.cidrap.umn.edu/news-perspective/2021/01/race-income-inequality-fuel-covid-disparities-us-counties#:~:text=They%20found%20that%20a%201.0,2.6%25%20rise%20in%20related%20deaths. Accessed December 8, 2022.

184 Operating in the Dark: The Gathering Crisis in Canada's Public Health Care System. Crowley, B., Zitner, D. 1999 https://www.researchgate.net/publication/237326223_Operating_in_the_Dark_The_Gathering_Crisis_in_Canada's_Public_Health_Care_System. Accessed December 8, 2022.

The Pandemic as a Model

The healthcare process kicks off with an individual patient having health complaints or attempting to maintain or manage health.

> **The initiating event for health care is the expression or uncovering of the problems and needs of patients**

Early in the pandemic, individuals found themselves feeling unwell with a puzzling array of symptoms that confused their doctors but indicated a possibly serious problem. Physicians examined these people and noted symptoms that included fever, cough, loss of the sense of smell and other neurological dysfunctions, breathing problems, malaise and distress. Many of these are common symptoms but usually not very distressing or present in lots of people at the same time. When physicians examined these people, they found alarming signs, including reduced lung function, low blood oxygen, blood clotting problems and neurological issues. These patients were seriously ill! It quickly became clear that an organism, soon discovered to be the novel SARS-CoV-2 virus that causes COVID-19, infected them. This was a diagnosis of a new viral disease.

> **The initial role of the physician is to listen to and examine the patient and to carry out the process of determining the cause of problems**

Worse still, the infected patients showed up at healthcare institutions in droves. This set off alarms regarding there being a significant Public Health problem, where a virus was spreading not only from an original source to people but from one person to another. Soon it became clear that it was a highly infectious and dangerous disease! This was a diagnosis of a disease that went beyond individual patients and was a Public Health emergency.

> **Sometimes many people are affected by the same problem, at which point the problem becomes an issue of Public Health**

Once it became likely that the disease was a virus and that it was infectious, i.e., was spreading from person to person, professionals quickly realized that they would need tests to determine if the virus had infected others, or if they might be victims of another problem, like Influenza. This necessitated a means of testing to confirm that the symptoms of many people had a common cause.

Food poisoning has been the classic example of a Public Health problem. With food poisoning, many people who have eaten the same food – usually contaminated with a bacterium – become sick with similar symptoms at the same time, then public health experts determine the causal agent. When the cause is known, for example infected lettuce or chicken, companies or agencies ask the sellers and consumers to discard the item.

Related to COVID-19, soon similar cases began to appear around the world and, eventually, the WHO determined that what was first a local spread – an epidemic – had become a pandemic: the virus had gone walk-about (in this case, 'fly-about') around the world. The local Public Health emergency had escalated to a global scale.

Testing to Find the Problem's Cause

The pandemic illustrates many aspects of testing.

> **Testing people to determine if they have the same cause of their problems as other people do is crucial and challenging, as all testing is imperfect**

First, SARS-CoV-2 was a novel virus; it was new to the world. So, researchers had to create a novel test that could reliably detect an infection with this virus, while ensuring that uninfected people were not labeled as infected. In other words, the test had to have high specificity and sensitivity. It had to indicate the true state of the patient. A false negative test result would allow an infected patient to remain in circulation and to infect others. The consequences of a false positive test result, on the other hand, would put an uninfected person into isolation and halt the person's work and travel. Regretfully, the first tests were quite poor. In some countries, like the United States, the initial testing of the population suffered from two major problems: (1) the test did not work properly because of technical problems, an incompatibility between chemicals used in the test, and (2) there were very, very few people with the disease at that time. This low prevalence meant that the test would need to have very high specificity in order to avoid labelling many healthy people as sick. With time, the tests became better and prevalence increased, so the results became more reliable.

The tests have improved dramatically since those first days. By now, many people have had COVID or are vaccinated. People are also taking the precautions they should take with any viral illness, regardless of whether they use the test or not.

In areas where the disease spread and infected many people, the tests were more useful, as it is easier to find needles in a haystack where there are lots of needles. In other areas, some tests, because they are imperfect, return results that are often misleading and interfere even today with post-pandemic management. It is interesting that few people, other than the most sophisticated healthcare experts, realize the true nature of testing, the problems that affect the usefulness of tests, and the importance of interpreting their results in the application context – low versus high prevalence environments. Tests can produce lots of false positive and false negative results with dire consequences for individuals and communities. To reiterate: false results include telling people they are sick, when they are not (a false positive) and telling people they are well when they are sick (a false negative).

> **There are many kinds of tests each for detecting a specific cause of problems and sometimes the tests mislead**

The problem of addressing the impacts of COVID-19 was further complicated by the introduction of tests that can detect if the person has had the infection previously. These are 'antibody' tests (the person's immune system produced antibodies to inactivate the virus), and, at the present time, these are less than perfectly reliable. Given this, the WHO has taken a stand against the idea of 'health passports', which would indicate that a person is purportedly immune to the virus because of having antibodies. Its reasoning is valid, as the current antibody and T-cell tests produce so many false positive results (saying that the person is immune to COVID-19), in effect giving them a pass to go out and get infected or infect others. Further, some people who are still infectious may have antibodies.[185] We have also learned that some people, despite being triple or quadruple vaxxed, could still harbor the infection, though much less likely to get very sick or die. One other point is that viruses often mutate and there may be a new variant circulating that the person's antibodies don't affect.

Clinical Treatment

Of course, the whole purpose of diagnosis is to discover what is wrong, if anything, and to

---

185 https://news.yahoo.com/can-you-have-coronavirus-antibodies-yet-still-be-contagious-100047820.html https://www.ncbi.nlm.nih.gov/pmc/articles/PMC7108922/. Accessed Feb. 10, 2023.

address the problem – that is, to treat it. A new kind of virus typically means that there needs to be a new kind of treatment, as it is unlikely that an already existing one will do the trick. Sometimes, though, we luck out and an existing treatment works against a novel infection. In the case of COVID-19, there were only a few lucky breaks.

Several existing treatments seemed to reduce some of the dramatic impacts of the virus. Medications, including steroids that reduce inflammation, and artificially ventilating patients, helped. Another treatment that seemed to be somewhat useful was the infusion of 'convalescent sera'.[186] These sera are the non-red cell, antibody carrying part of the blood (plasma) from previously infected but recovered patients. So far at least, these treatments have, at best, helped some patients recover more quickly and seem to have reduced mortality. Therapies helped control and reduced the impact od the disease much as antiretroviral treatments have helped manage HIV. One antiviral therapy is Paxlovid, which people can take by mouth.[187] In addition, there are others.[188] Regretfully, as the virus evolves, its newer variants often become less vulnerable to these interventions.

> **Diagnosis, which is the determination of the cause or origin of the patient's problems, Informs interventions intended to address them in effective ways**

Accepting and being confident of new treatments requires that we first test them on volunteers or as last-ditch (compassionate) efforts to save a patient. We do this to learn if the drug is safe and effective. The testing of treatments should be on people similar to those who will eventually receive the treatment. Therefore, testing should include many age groups and people with a variety of health characteristics. In other words, test subjects should be representative of the general population.

> **New treatments must first be tested and shown to be safe and effective and produce more benefit than harm**

Public Health Treatment

The ultimate 'treatments' in the case of a pandemic like COVID-19 include vaccines, interventions or other agents that either prevent infection or dramatically reduce effects in a protected person. Absent the ability to prevent infection, isolation, quarantine and distancing can keep infected people away from others so they cannot transmit the infection.

Because COVID-19 had not previously infected people – at least as far as we know – there was no pre-existing vaccine. The game has changed with the availability of effective vaccines against COVID. They seem to reduce the chance of getting infected and lower the severity of infection in vaccinated people who become infected. Success here has meant not only creating the vaccine but manufacturing it in vast volume, so it was available to and accepted by billions of people, as the whole world was at risk. The problem is that vaccines in the past have taken take many years to develop and some, like for HIV, have eluded the best efforts of science.

186 The convalescent sera option for containing COVID-19 - PMC (nih.gov)Casadevall A, Pirofski LA. The convalescent sera option for containing COVID-19. J Clin Invest. 2020 Apr 1;130(4):1545-1548. doi: 10.1172/JCI138003. PMID: 32167489; PMCID: PMC7108922. https://pubmed.ncbi.nlm.nih.gov/32167489/. Accessed December 8, 2022.

187 https://www.fda.gov/news-events/press-announcements/coronavirus-covid-19-update-fda-authorizes-first-oral-antiviral-treatment-covid-19. Accessed December 8, 2022.

188 https://www.cdc.gov/coronavirus/2019-ncov/your-health/treatments-for-severe-illness.html. Accessed December 8, 2022.

Vaccines are not perfect in terms of protecting people and, very rarely, some people can experience occasionally serious harm.

> **Scientists must develop safe and effective treatments, industry must manufacture them, people must accept them, they must be widely and affordably available and people must accept them**

The world had not previously responded in a sufficiently adaptive way to dealing with novel – especially highly contagious – viruses by having or developing and widely deploying testing and contact tracing mechanisms, ubiquitous quarantining and critical care facilities, and therapeutics and vaccines in a timely fashion. The evolution of at least partially effective responses has produced some basis for future pandemic prevention, better management and treatment. To achieve this related to COVID-19, nations backed corporations and put test development and deployment, the identification of therapeutics and vaccine development into very high gear by advancing billions of dollars in at-risk funding. Laboratories began early manufacturing of vaccines and did rapid trials to test that they worked and did not harm people. One would hope that what we did in response to COVID-19 was not a one-off approach but rather that agencies will create durable structures that can promptly respond to future challenges.

We must realize that this radical approach may not always work. It may be that developing vaccines for certain viruses will continue to be challenging, and researchers will sometimes fail or it will take decades to develop them. It may also be that we develop vaccines that cause other problems, like intolerable side effects or even infections. This has happened with many vaccines, including one that was eventually successful, the polio vaccine. However, modern

information technologies and techniques make it easier to track the benefits and harms of any novel (or existing) intervention. In the meantime, people are not powerless; they can use personal measures to reduce viral spread.

One important hope that is now on the horizon is the creation of 'universal vaccines', though these may be limited to impacting one family of viruses, such as the Corona Viruses of which SARS-CoV-2 is a member.[189]

> **Health care, ultimately, involves personal responsibility**

Social or Personal Intervention —

Perhaps the most interesting aspect of the pandemic has been the recognition by scientists and knowledgeable people regarding what individuals can do to prevent infection. From the very beginning of the pandemic, Public Health professionals communicated widely and often that excellent handwashing hygiene would prevent virus on surfaces from entering the body. The other even more crucial intervention was 'social distancing' (better stated as 'physical distancing') and the wearing of masks when distancing was not possible. Some countries have long histories of mask-wearing, which thwarted the virus's transfer from person-to-person. Masks are particularly important because COVID is a respiratory virus – especially affecting the respiratory tract and the lungs. But not all masks are equal.

The special masks healthcare workers wore (called 'N95 respirators') largely prevented the inhalation of the virus. The purpose of masks used by the general public is the reduction of viral transmission from an infected person to a noninfected person. Unfortunately, this simple, inexpensive and fairly effective intervention became a political issue in the United States and some other

189 https://covid19.nih.gov/news-and-stories/exploring-new-approach-universal-vaccines-against-covid-19. Accessed December 8, 2022.

countries during the COVID pandemic and the consequence has been hundreds of thousands of additional infections as leaders attempted to reopen the economy and return to a degree of social normalcy. Many, wishing to make a political or personal statement, rejected this almost cosmetic intervention in favor of infection and even death. Think of that! Multitudes of people have donned ridiculous hats or scarves that some fashionista wore to an event – an action of zero social value. However, some of those same people rejected a personal undertaking that might have saved countless lives. Humanity is *weird!*

Misinformation is a serious threat generally in health care. However, in a pandemic it can be as dangerous as the contagious organism and can spread (no pun intended) virally nationwide and worldwide

---

An important issue in an epidemic or pandemic is ensuring that healthcare professionals are properly equipped and protected

---

We must become aware that health is crucial for a dynamic economy, a functioning society and the comfort and function of all people

---

The Societal Aspects of Health —

The story of masks is a significant example of the importance of the social dimension of health. However, it is not the only example. The pandemic points out several other social issues:

Health is significantly influenced by a person's context: social and physical environment, economic status, and nutrition

---

1. The behavior of each of us affects both our own health and the health of those around us. The COVID-19 pandemic makes it clear that there are often simple, personal interventions that can reduce the need for more invasive and expensive interventions.

2. Our priorities and the weights we place on various aspects of our lives can dramatically affect both our health and the health of others. How important is it to go to a bar, attend a rave, yell and scream at a political convention in the midst of epidemic infections versus protecting ourselves and others? However, some societal interventions, particularly related to keeping kids out of schools, had significant unintended consequences; post-pandemic evaluation revealed that many students had lost ground in their educations.

3. The importance we place on our and our fellow humans' living conditions, economic status, access to food, health care, communications and a supportive social milieu is nowhere near what it needs to be. The poor, people of color, the homeless, the physically impaired, the elderly and the uninsured all find themselves ghettoized when it comes to good health and adequate health care.

4. How we choose our government and who our leaders are can determine into which group we fall, the living or the dead.

5. The people with whom we communicate and intermingle can impact our belief systems, undermine our trust of experts and their guidance, and it can affect the validity of the information we ingest.

6. The societal investment and intellectual capital we invest in the full length and breadth of the health system have not only dramatic impacts on the quality of

life but also on our economic livelihoods. It is high time to realize that adequate investment in health, health education and disease prevention and promotion, health care, Public Health, interagency cooperation and coordination and leadership is crucial not only related to health but also related to the GDP.[190]

The Pandemic as a Test

Back in the financial crisis that began in the first decade of the 21st century, the Congress of the United States recognized that the banking system had problems. The result was that Congress mandated the application of 'stress tests' to determine if banks were viable and stable or needed to alter their financial state. COVID-19 has been a stress test on the entire healthcare complex! What's worse, the healthcare system and its leadership FAILED the test! The existing systems weren't resilient and they didn't have the tools or capacity to respond to this type of problem and deal with the surges in demand for testing, treatments and care. In the United States alone, over 1,000,000 (1 million) people died and an estimated 6.6 million succumbed globally… and both numbers are likely underestimates! Compare that to the 'only' 300,000 Americans who died in World War 2.

> Sickness and disease can and have challenged entire nations indicating that healthcare, especially Public Health, is a national security issue

COVID-19 tested every healthcare institution and forced them to adapt to massive influxes of very sick patients. It tested care providers and made it clear that they must be able to secure materials to protect themselves so that they can help their patients. COVID-19 also tested inter-organizational cooperation and coordination, as well as local, state, provincial and federal governments. In fact, COVID-19 tested and continues to test the world's approach to health care! The virus showed us that pretty much every needed aspect of the healthcare system was lacking, compromised or vulnerable.

Only personal heroism carried care providers through the crisis.

They were indeed heroic! The truth is that they had to be heroic or they and their patients would have died in even greater numbers! Health professionals, unlike soldiers, enter their professions to help people – not possibly kill them or die themselves. Unlike soldiers, we do not train healthcare workers to accept mortal danger as a part of their duties. However, COVID-19 killed an estimated 115,000 of them worldwide[191] and yet they still placed themselves in harm's way. They exhibited the highest measure of bravery and, in doing so, helped countless thousands. The key point is that we should not expect that ultimate sacrifice! The failures of leadership and the system inflicted that on them. We must never let that happen again!

> The life and viability of each of our lives depends to a significant extent on our health, health care-related decisions, and the quality and effectiveness of healthcare and other services that affect the social determinants of health

---

190 https://macdonaldlaurier.ca/measuring-health-managing-health-care-routinely-pandemics-david-zitner-inside-policy/. Accessed December 8, 2022.

191 https://www.who.int/news/item/20-10-2021-health-and-care-worker-deaths-during-covid-19. Accessed December 8, 2022.

Thinking About
the Unthinkable[192] ——————————

Our final thought is rather depressing. We do not apologize.

What would the healthcare system and the population of the world be like if, instead of a viral pandemic, the threat had been widespread devastation, death, loss of services and radioactive fallout from a local or global thermonuclear war? By comparison, COVID "ain't nothin'"![193] [194]

It's hard to imagine why we maintain millions of weapons of self-annihilation having seen what even a nano-sized virus can do!

---

192 https://www.economist.com/briefing/2020/06/25/the-world-should-think-better-about-catastrophic-and-existential-risks. Accessed December 8, 2022.

193 https://www.atomicarchive.com/resources/documents/effects/wenw/introduction.html. Accessed December 8, 2022.

194 https://en.wikipedia.org/wiki/Nuclear_holocaust. Accessed Feb. 10, 2023.

APPENDIX 1: ——— Thinking Big: The Humongous Body and Mind and Their Impacts on Information and Care Policy

KEYWORDS: Humongous Body, Humongous Mind, Policy, Chardin, Social Media, Misinformation, Disinformation, White Lie Packaging, Intentional Misrepresentation, Mind-altering Information, Manufactured Mis-evidence, Saturation Mis-information, Ignorance Tolerance, Misinformation Epidemic, Misinformation Pandemic, Information Fit, Misinformation Proof, Peer Review, Questions to Ask

ABSTRACT: Many have begun to recognize the nature and effects of misinformation and disinformation so ably promulgated by manipulators via the Internet, the Web and social media. Social networks on the Internet have, in reality, effected what we call the 'Humongous Mind' – the interconnected ensemble of all human minds, enabled by a neural-like network that can both improve and endanger global mental health. On an immediate basis, despite the extant danger, it may be – like Civil Defence in the 1950s – that all most of us can do is to be careful and skeptical, limiting ourselves to a few authoritative sources of information and communications, as well as a trusted community of contacts, and sticking to those. Our global approach to the health of the Humongous Body is primitive, but we have not yet evolved any means for the care of the Humongous Mind. Worse, we have an environment that misinformation and disinformation infest, and where incredibly efficient technologies assure its dissemination. This environment provides a digitally enhanced universe populated with abundant bad actors who want to negatively affect our thinking, feeling and behavior. We posit the need for a 'conscience' for the Humongous Mind that policy and enforcement might provide.

Introduction: the Problem of Misinformation in Electronic Media – a Public Health Problem -

Many people have begun to recognize the nature and effects of misinformation and disinformation so ably promulgated by manipulators via the Internet, the Web and social media. Most can sense that manipulated media are dangerous to everyone, young and old, sophisticated or naïve because we all depend on the media to form an understanding of reality – what is actually happening around us. How can civil society more deeply understand and moderate the dangers of misinformation?

The Clear and Present Danger ——

Internet-based electronic communications facilities and social networks are valuable because they connect us tightly to each other, allowing us to share useful and interesting facts and thoughts and learn about our local and global situation. Unfortunately, modern communications technologies also enable serious social pathology in ways not experienced before.

Social networks on the Internet have, in reality, effected what we call the 'Humongous Mind', the interconnected ensemble of all human minds, enabled by a neural-like network that can both improve and endanger global mental health.

About 70 years ago, Teilhard de Chardin[195], an idealistic thinker, defined an interesting concept: that humans will evolve into a *"living skin of the Earth"*. As a Jesuit priest and philosopher, he saw this from a religious viewpoint. However, it isn't much of a stretch to recognize that this kind of change has begun.

Sure, we individual beings were already physically interconnected – made possible by transportation technology. We have called the result of that the 'Humongous Body'. Now, though, our neural-like technology enables an even deeper interconnectedness of our minds: the Humongous Mind. If we do not recognize the significant issues engendered by tight, nearly instantaneous mental interconnectedness, we will not appreciate new failure modes, not to mention new opportunities. Both exist, with the result of both unwanted devastating social disruptions as well as dramatic and worthwhile social benefits.

Regretfully, this interconnected super-system of minds lacks a monitoring, management and care system to assure its value and prevent or treat the pathologies it engenders. It lacks a

conscience. This means that our understanding and care of the Humongous Mind is in a state like that our understanding and care of our bodies were in before the advent of modern medical science.

There has been much discussion around Internet communications policy to guide the regulation of content on social networks and manage the effects that advanced software, like Artificial Intelligence-based algorithms, can have. Regulation must have clearly stated purposes and goals, so we can determine whether new regulations or behaviors are helping or harming. Before any of us can consider regulation and policy, however, we must more deeply understand why we need it and what outcomes we must achieve.

Our Message ———————

We urgently require policy related to communications content and processes that preserves the positive aspects of modern technologies but minimizes their extraordinarily dangerous negative impacts. We have called this the 'conscience' of the Humongous Mind. However, this policy is challenging to formulate – especially in face of the freedom of speech – and almost insuperable to apply and enforce. It is a challenge like the one we have faced and continue to confront in nuclear arms control. This new threat, though different, also has the potential of immense societal disruption, already exemplified in political divisions, which society will almost certainly increasingly and more devastatingly experience – that is, unless we take steps to intervene.

On an immediate basis, despite the extant danger, it may be that – like Civil Defence in the 1950s – all most of us can do is to be careful and skeptical, limiting ourselves to a few authoritative sources of information and communications, as well as a trusted community of contacts, and sticking to those. We can at the very least "information proof" ourselves,

---

195 https://www.britannica.com/biography/Pierre-Teilhard-de-Chardin. Accessed Feb. 10, 2023.

which we address below. This is like what we face in addressing our personal health: we protect ourselves from sickness through proper nutrition, becoming and remaining fit and being careful even when promoters encourage poor health behaviors!

Right now, for the Humongous Mind and, to some extent, even for the Humongous Body – as countries have neglected Public Health (through underfunding, shuttering laboratories, failing to invest in information technology and reducing professional resources) – it's "patient, heal thyself". Our global approach to the health of the Humongous Body is primitive, but we have not yet evolved any means for the care of the Humongous Mind. Worse, we have an environment that is ridden with misinformation and disinformation supported by the technologies that incredibly efficiently connect us and abundant bad actors who want to negatively affect our thinking, feeling and behavior.

Given this situation, we must at least develop methods to manage what we access and what or who can access us. We need to find means of inhibiting the exchange of fake news, "alternative facts", external interference and the hacking of communications content, as these all impact how we think, feel and act.

Human beings have not, after more than 70 years, evolved a means of fully protecting the world from a thermonuclear disaster. However, we do have some arms control measures that have kept the planet relatively safe, even if on the edge. Perhaps national policy and internation treaties regarding misinformation are partial answers for toxic content, malevolent interference and corrupt informers.

Though we are individual beings, we are globally united physically, like it or not. Next, though we have individual minds, our thinking is becoming more and more interlocked globally. We are all threatened by bad information and deliberate interference with our thinking. Agents who want to mess with my mind, who may not even know me, now have a direct channel into it. If I am not 'information-proofed', they can succeed and determine the course of my life or even my death.

Potential Dangers Created or Enhanced by Communications Technology and Social Media ——

The following represent the major characteristics of our existing information and communications infrastructure:

1. Universal and ubiquitous access to and sourcing of content (anyone can input and access information). This gives everyone, including deliberate manipulators, access to our minds.

2. Almost instantaneous access to information regardless of source, quality and validity. We receive and read information before we have much time to detect or consider problems or threats.

3. The ability to capture usage (including specific content exchanged) and user ID and demographic information and apply this information to influence individuals and populations. This enables almost closed-loop mind control, a perfect example being the reinforcement of suicidal ideation.

4. The ability to determine recipients' information wants, needs, preferences and identities and reinforce them, with or without their permission – as well as the difficulty in opting out. Companies quietly trap people.

5. The use of algorithms – AI and other software – to analyze what users do, seek and request, and then respond. This is like having a constant online alter ego, not necessarily a good one.

6. A dearth of information content and source quality review and certification agents.

7. Minimal societal interest in and means to deal with the pathologies that result.

8. The substitution of direct discourse with affect-suppressing virtual interaction. In this, we lose a capability that at least helps us detect deceit and attempts at exploitation.

9. The ability to create hard-to-detect visual and auditory fakes. Manipulators can paint their version of reality on the inside of our eyeballs, and it looks and sounds real.

10. The policy and regulation vacuum: minimal or no information- and communications-related policy. Commercial and political interests seem to inhibit rule making.

11. The policing vacuum: minimal detection of violations and enforcement of even the negligible existing policies. Surely, we need some means of detecting violations and enforcing regulations.

The Kind of Policy that Can Help

We recognize that addressing the need for policy to deal with these problems requires international as well as national agreements and that it will be challenging to develop. Nonetheless, there is a need for action to counter the dangers, though we again find ourselves recognizing the need for technology policy after the proverbial horse has escaped the barn.

We are aware that many have made suggestions regarding the control of content and its dissemination. However, the threat to the freedom of speech and the fact that this is exactly what autocratic governments do to constrain their citizens' thinking, should put pause to interventions like these. We do offer

that the following as the kinds of actions could possibly help (no priority intended):

> All information and communications should be meta-tagged at least with an identifiable source, date and other information in addition to standard email tracking tags. Ideally, Internet servers' software could flag messages with inconsistencies among tags (such as the sender's stated email address and the actual email origin) as 'from a questionable source', so receivers can choose to accept, ignore, delete or block the sender. This could also allow receivers to identify the actual sender. If sellers can use software to influence buying, we can also use it to protect receivers.

> Communities can consider incorporating the ability to recognize and delay distribution of communications tagged as indicating threats of violence or other harms. This would inhibit rapid initiation of riots and violent uprisings. The software can notify senders of the delay.

> We can write privacy and other related policies in simple and clear terms, providing an opt-in (not just opt-out) opportunity that must be regularly reapproved.

> A trusted NGO agency(ies) can review algorithms and inform users of the algorithms' purpose, mode of operation, potential benefits and harms, as well as any potential violations of regulations and laws. Furthermore, every user should be able to opt-in to and regularly reapprove the application of an algorithm to them.

> Public education must address apathy by informing sources and users of the issues, dangers, potential solutions, policies and penalties. Consider the creation

of a Computer Drivers License[196] like that available in Europe, extended to deal with the matters we have addressed. Educators could be offer this in early school years and in continuing education programs. It could provide education on the interpersonal and societal impacts of the technology, including the mental impacts on non-face-to-face communications and the rapid spread and danger of mis/disinformation.

> Governmental and non-governmental agencies should collaborate and cooperate related to developing the evidence base for policy development, policy promulgation and regulation.

> We should empower our communities to enforce policy and address violations.

We are not naïve regarding the issues associated with interventions like these. However, some advance in this direction would be superior to what we are experiencing in terms of the personal, societal and even global impacts of the status quo. We must recognize that societal conflict, disruption and death are the predictable effects of misinformation and disinformation

Now we will turn our attention to developing an understanding of the nature of information, misinformation and disinformation, as well as their impacts on the Humongous Mind.

Information in the Anthropocene Era

In the past, the sources of information were fewer and more easily traceable to a credible or dubious source. There were malicious informers, like authoritarian leaders, that propagated information to manipulate their captive populations. However, ordinary people had limited access to the channels of communication, and the limitations of the available media inhibited rapid replication and dissemination. Then, as now, bad actors could publish a deceitful book, broadcast propaganda, circulate fraudulent articles or communicate false gossip over the telephone or in the visual or print media. However, the reach of an individual was limited, and the effort and cost of dissemination were onerous. Now, social media, the Web, the Internet and other tools offer a 'bully pulpit', and anyone can reach almost everyone.

Types of Misinformation

Misinformation comes in many forms. Perhaps recognizing the face of evil will help avoid it.

Misinformation can be **Innocent Misstatements**, garbled facts, unintentional misquotes, the biproducts of confusion or the misunderstood conclusions of a study. Sometimes it can be an opinion twisted by bias, or a topic 'spun' by a politician. These are largely unavoidable artifacts of ordinary human beings. Generally, they are not malicious, though often manipulative. Wondering about validity should be our normal response.

Misinformation can also be the attractive packaging of a commercial product. Let's call that **White Lie Packaging**, intended to catalyze purchasing with little or no consideration of the product's helpfulness or harmfulness. Sometimes this might be relatively innocent, like claiming that a product ablates wrinkles. Other times this can have lethal effects; cigarette advertising is the perfect example.

A greater problem is **Disinformation: Intentional Misrepresentations** from someone motivated to pervert another's thinking, feeling or acting to serve an interest. A

---

196 The International Computer Driver's License certification is a globally recognised ICT and digital literacy qualification showing that people have a set of recognized computer skills. The European Computer Driving Licence (ECDL) is a Europe-wide qualification in basic computer skills. If you have passed ECDL, employers know you have the skills to carry out the main tasks on a computer. The ECDL is the first qualification in personal computing skills to be recognised throughout the European Union. https://en.wikipedia.org/wiki/European_Computer_Driving_Licence. Accessed Feb. 10, 2023.

more innocent version is when a politician or braggard denigrates an opponent. There can be, however, more nasty effects at the extreme of the spectrum. Let us look at these varieties of maliciousness.

Consider deliberate **Mind-altering Misinformation** – the information equivalent of psychoactive drugs. People promulgate it to cause others to think, feel or decide in certain ways or to ideologically bias them. This is usually at the receivers' expense and can injure them. One example is "alternative facts" to influence targeted populations to, for instance, ignore political malfeasance or visual evidence.

Another malicious intervention is the fabrication of false information: **Manufactured Mis-evidence**. This is like creating a fake medication, and can involve promoting false concepts, misrepresentation of test results or manufacturing of falsified data. Fraudsters do this to benefit themselves financially or otherwise. Volkswagen's fraud regarding diesel engines is a good example.[197]

A common source of misinformation is people who traffic in conspiracy theories. These include non-scientific theories of disease or its treatment, often backed by claims that reputable science ignores their theories because they undermine mainstream producers' profitability. Some harbor misconceptions or aberrant beliefs, or they may just be trying to fool us. They include claims that vaccinations cause Autism or include computer chips – this might give people a chip for their shoulders if they don't already have one. Theories sometimes mix in genuine science.

Perhaps the most malignant forms of misinformation are **Saturation Misinformation** and the facilitation of **Ignorance Tolerance**. Governments that control all information can do the former. But agents can be silent about or downplay information about genuine dangers.

Some have kept the toxic effects Lead in the water system[198] or radioactive Radon gas[199] under wraps. This leaves people unaware and unconcerned – under a 'mental anesthetic'. The lack of information is the ultimate threat, as we are not aware and we unknowingly share our ignorance. Worse than communicable, we are already infected!

Misinformation Epidemics involve the spread of false or biased information within a region and **Misinformation Pandemics** circle the world. The infectiousness of misinformation varies enormously based on its source (e.g., a President or religious leader), the transmission method (for example, the Internet) and the susceptibility of the population (like people seeking support of their own biases).

Misinformation is a Transmissable Malignant Disease

Virtually everyone today has concern about the environment, realizing that pollution can cause or potentiate illnesses, including cancers and even death. Worse, its effects can be slow and insidious. Some are also awakening to the realization that there is another kind of toxic emission – misinformation – that originates from fellow humans and they communicate it person-to-person through their eyes and ears. A clear and present danger, it can poison, cause societal dysfunction and result in death. It can be a weapon of mass distraction or destruction, especially during a pandemic. It is contagious, needing no direct contact, its vector being communications systems. We are all vulnerable and there is no 100%-effective vaccine.

197 https://www.bbc.com/news/business-34324772. Accessed Feb. 10, 2023.
198 https://www.nrdc.org/stories/flint-water-crisis-everything-you-need-know. Accessed Feb. 10, 2023.
199 http://www.waterkeeper.ca/blog/2016/11/8/what-you-need-to-know-about-the-port-hope-area-radioactive-waste-cleanup. Accessed Feb. 10, 2023.

The Treatment: Dealing with Misinformation

Developing effective interventions to deal with misinformation is challenging and may need to be planet-level! As often is the case, the best intervention would be a prepared – think: 'vaccinated' – mind, high quality sources and critical thinking. Given the plethora of bizarre sources, that may be it!

We have become an information society, built on agencies, companies and media that are information dependent and copious information sources with wide-band communication channels. The potential for misinformation is enormous and easily reaches into our homes and our individual lives. The Internet provides embedded, direct and efficient channels for misinformation. It is naïve to think that we only get correct information or that just some of it is wrong or a little off and won't harm us! Almost any misinformation is a danger, and its effects can be subtle and delayed. Think heavy metals in the water supply as an analogy. Worse still is the dearth of high-quality curated information.

Health Promotion and Prevention for the Individual Mind

Right now, we live in a public policy and enforcement vacuum. However, individuals can take some steps to avoid Misinformation Disease and its pathological mental effects. This is not easy, because information is the basis for virtually everything we think, feel, decide and do. A preventive to the impacts of misinformation is to become **Information Fit** or **Misinformation Proofed**:

1. **Find and use reliable and authoritative information sources.** Undertake to select information from reputable sources, preferably vetted by agents, organizations or agencies that we trust. Admittedly, determining trustworthiness is challenging, as we may mistakenly depend on officials or organizations that have ulterior motives or that by default misinform us.

2. **Ask questions and be sure to get cogent answers** especially when of consequence, even regarding the information coming from purportedly reliable sources. An important question is: Does what I have heard, read or seen make sense? Does it comport with what I already know? If not, look further. This is especially important for people immersed in misinformation and judging new information based on that. Going afield of usual sources and considering others is crucial.

3. **Determine if information has been peer reviewed and by whom**. That is a crucial check. Peer review (the evaluation of the methods, results and interpretation of research by qualified experts) is the 'good housekeeping seal of approval'. Even this is not a sure thing, as scientists sometimes self-serve or support friends. 'Expert' is often a self-awarded title. Perhaps the best solution is to realize this and consider several 'expert' assertions in the light of item 7 below.

4. **Crosscheck or triangulate multiple sources** – trusting only one source or evaluator is risky.

5. **Decide if the claim is verifiable.** Can I become knowledgeable and use scientific thinking to get to the same point? It is the personal acceptance test.

6. **Always harbor healthy skepticism!** Never say "uncle" to information or a source! Only trust information of consequence after you verify. Foster a doubt even if assured and be curious to find the truth, if and when that is important to deciding or acting – often humans must function in the face of ambiguity.

7. **If unsure, we must determine what we require to mediate between**

conflicting claims. When there is no way to test claims versus counter claims, they become opinion only.

The National Institutes of Health has published "How to Evaluate Health Information on the Internet: Questions and Answers".[200] The document suggests asking key questions paraphrased with additions here:

1. **Who runs the website?** Is this a reliable source or might it deliberately or inadvertently provide misinformation or disinformation?

2. **Who pays for it?** Is the source trying to influence our buying behavior? This objective can cause the originator to 'spin' the information or fail to state the whole truth.

3. **What is the original source of the information?** Is it opinion dressed up to look authoritative? Good information will be based on scientific studies. However, recognize that that some studies on which we might depend and have consequences are themselves biased, self-serving, fraudulent or otherwise unreliable.

4. **Was the website information reviewed by an expert based on genuine evidence?** Most of the material on the Web is not in any way reviewed or certified by impartial organizations. Wikipedia, for example, is widely depended on. Is Wikipedia information referenced to support statements? Some assertions are opinions and subject to change by other participants, while other content may be observable facts.

5. **How will the website use the fact that you searched for the information?** Is the website just bait to capture information about you? You may not be able to determine this prospectively. You will probably find out if ads bombard you afterward.

Answering these questions is challenging, often time consuming and may be beyond many of us. Even answering them will not guarantee misinformation-proofing, but this may be the best we can do as individuals. Realize that even respected and trusted scientists have gotten things wrong[201] and inadvertently misinformed their peers and the public. We all need our own Index of Suspicion!

Probably the best way to approach information is to consider it a hypothesis that, if not disproved, stands as the best we can do…until and if we or someone else disprove it.

It is best if we recognize that Web information is like brackish water – a mix of fresh and saltwater like in a tidal river – some of it potable but some not! Anyone, with any kind of interest or for any reason, can place information there to achieve the source's positive or negative objectives. Nothing prevents disturbed or manipulative agents from polluting it with toxic info-effluent. And anyone can search for anything: ways to kill, make bombs, concoct poisons, perpetrate fraud and just about any nightmarish purpose. It is the ultimate resource and medium for bad actors.

Fortunately, the Web also hosts vast amounts of valuable information. Only the searching skills, critical thinking ability and good intentions can assure that is what we get. We need to information-proof ourselves (and our children) – street-proofing for life on the information superhighway!

---

200 https://ods.od.nih.gov/HealthInformation/How_To_Evaluate_Health_Information_on_the_Internet_Questions_and_Answers.aspx. Accessed December 8, 2022.
201 Fermi and transuranics: https://vimeo.com/143066365. Accessed Feb. 10, 2023.

A Model for Understanding the Potential and Dangers of Social Networking ———————

THE CONNECTED WORLD

Most have recognized that local, national and international transportation have enabled us to be more socially connected than ever before. COVID-19 pandemic and Climate Change make it clear that even more so we are biologically connected. The Internet, especially social media (Facebook, Twitter and the like), has made us informationally connected. However, mass political and societal disturbance – such as conspiracy theory-driven, highly emotionally charged and even violent disagreement – shows that our technology enables a deeper, more pervasive and potentially pathological connection we have not previously faced: Our minds are being 'virtually connected' in near real time. For some, this has diminished, inhibited or even eliminated independent thought and consideration, substituting dependence on echo chambers and information sources curated to support biases. Analogically, we now have a long distance 'neurological' connection that does draw us closer together, but also enables mass-thinking pathologies with which we are struggling. Star Trek had its Borg[202], and we confront a similar future.

So far, no one has suggested a term that encompasses all of humanity. Using words like "The Collective" is a possibility, but we use the term 'Humongous Being' to recognize that we face problems as if we all are one.

The Human Being ———————

Each human being has a physical body and a mind emerging from the brain's function. The purpose of healthcare is to support the comfort, function and lifespan of the human being. That purpose should apply to **each** human being, as well as to the **ensemble** of all humans. **John Donne wrote: "No man is an Island".**[203] That poem recognizes that we are

and must be connected and integrated, especially when it comes to our health. Pandemics make that obvious.

The Human Being's Body ———————

Our individual bodies comprise organs, like the brain, heart and lungs, that perform necessary life functions. These organs work together in systems, like the digestive system comprising the mouth, esophagus, stomach and intestines. Bodily organs interconnect and intercommunicate with each other through the blood vessels and nerves. So, the body is a system of systems working together.

The healthy human body has healthy organs with healthy interconnections among them. Of course, disease, deprivation or trauma can narrow or block blood vessels, injure or sever nerves. The result will be that organs, organ systems or the entire body suffers impairment, damage or death. Spinal injuries, for example, can cause paralysis because the damage interrupts the connection between the brain and the limbs.

Medical professionals and healthcare centers are two of our answers to problems with the components of the body. Another answer is our own efforts to maintain physical fitness and adequate nutrition.

The Human Being's Mind ———————

Just as the health of the body can suffer, so too can the health of the mind.

Disorders of the brain can affect the mind. For instance, Alzheimer's disease can impair or destroy a person's memory. Also, people might be born with structural problems of the brain. Life context also influences the mind, so mental health issues can develop in the absence of disordered biology.

However, there are other and even more ubiquitous causes of problems of the mind:

---

202 https://fr.wikipedia.org/wiki/Borg_(Star_Trek). Accessed Feb. 10, 2023.
203 https://web.cs.dal.ca/~johnston/poetry/island.html. Accessed Feb. 10, 2023.

disorders of thinking, feeling and behavior. Nothing may be wrong with the brain, but thinking can be disturbed. Normally the mind works well enough to enable us to cope. However, sometimes our environment, situation or those around us affect the function of our minds – abuse, catastrophes and disinformation can do that. Disorders of the mind can seriously impair our thinking, feeling and functioning.

Correcting the effects of problems like these is the objective of mental health care – we, those around us, or professional therapists try to help us to maintain or improve our mental healthiness.

The Humongous Body

We have coined the term 'Humongous Body' – the 'Body' of bodies that inhabit the globe – to represent our physical interconnectedness.

We may forget that we are not just individuals, but members of social, societal, philosophical and even larger groups, some spanning beyond national or geographical boundaries. We each are living parts of the entire population of our planet.

The 'Humongous Body' expression recognizes that we are all parts of a system, the amalgamated system of all human beings. As we individually comprise systems, so the population of the Earth is a super-system of systems, comprising all humans. Governments unite us into one kind of human super-system. But these are loosely coupled super-systems that an election, a war, or another intervention can change. The Humongous Body is a tighter and more robust super-system that unites us all, regardless of our political and other identities. The Humongous Body comprises groups of people. Some grow crops, others manufacture products, and still others deliver things to us, teach us how to think about and do things, and finance these activities. Today, we find ourselves dependent on others for our resources, products and services. We have

fulfilled Donne's prophesy: people are no longer islands.

The interconnections among the components of the Humongous Body are ships, trains, cars and planes, on the waterways, railroads, highways and airways that support movement.

So, we find ourselves in a physically interconnected and interdependent world, where people thrive or perish based on that interconnectedness and our recognition of interdependence. What's more, any problem — any 'pathology' – in one group or area of the world can seriously impact people in other areas. Infectious diseases make this clear. However, pathology in our interdependence can also cause shortages of computer chips or the scarcity of essential minerals. Production in one area serves the needs of other areas and the selling of those materials supports the economy of the supplier and the purchasers. If the various parts of the Humongous Body interact productively and each part plays its role, the Humongous Body is healthy. If parts fail, the whole Humongous Body suffers.

We want to illustrate that our interdependence globally is much like the interdependence we have on our own organ systems.

The Humongous Mind

As the human being comprises a body and a mind, so does the Humongous Being.

Whole countries operate under common (mental) understandings, which they elucidate in constitutions or philosophies of government. That is the result of multiple minds choosing to coordinate their thinking, behave according to certain commonly held principles and have feelings of pride in their nation or heritage. We all function like this in our own minds related to our personal lives.

We are not asserting a strict correspondence between how an individual's mind functions and how the Humongous Mind functions, but rather we want to indicate that there IS a Humongous Mind. That Humongous

Mind spans, links and unites groups with certain beliefs, such as religions, countries, political blocs, and, ultimately, the entire world. An example of a global 'thought' of the Humongous Mind is global awareness and concern regarding climate change or a belief in a basic right to happiness.

The Humongous Mind has interconnections much like those between the components of the brain or the other components of the body.

For the Humongous Mind, the interconnections are communications systems, including the media, telephones, e-mail, and social software. The Humongous Mind has recently evolved a radical kind of interconnectivity – the Internet – that enables universal sharing of individual thinking.

The advent of social networks is shocking! Suddenly, we can virtually instantaneously share thinking among dispersed groups. Before, that was far more difficult, expensive and slow. It's as if the Humongous Mind has evolved to the full human level.

The Pathology of the Humongous Mind ————

> **Problems - pathology - can emerge in the individual's mind; so can they in the Humongous Mind.**

There are many pathologies of the Humongous Mind. 'Societal Alzheimer's' is a Humongous Mind pathology where we forget history or past mistakes or inhibit access to information about the past. This is already the case in places that ignore the repeated holocausts humanity has endured.

Another pathology can be 'Societal Delusion' caused by people perverting others in their social network with mistaken ideation – misinformation. Hearing ideation repeatedly can reinforce our personal thinking. So can misinformation affect the Humongous

Mind via our networks. Algorithms can make it worse.

What we might refer to as 'Social Psychoses' of the Humongous Mind can occur when manipulators create weird beliefs – like conspiracy theories – or fraudsters promote fake data or news.

Every other mental problem can afflict the Humongous Mind. Masses of people can become depressed, can enter a bipolar state by being whipsawed from one way of thinking to another. We can find every behavioral and feeling problem replicated at the mass level.

Misinformation is the primary cause of disorders of the Humongous Mind. We spelled out the nature and some of the detailed effects of misinformation and disinformation.

Care for the Humongous Body and the Humongous Mind ————

When it comes to Humongous Health Care, there is some bad news. The recent pandemic demonstrated that the healthcare system for the Humongous Body – the 'Public Health System' – is weak and dysfunctional, having been systematically under-resourced and only an asset of wealthy countries. Information about infections was not properly communicated, nor were infections expeditiously detected and traced. Only heroic efforts enabled the development of vaccines and therapeutics. Public Health had withered despite the efforts of the WHO. The result: hundreds of millions became sick, many requiring hospitalization, and millions died. Locally, Public Health Care is poor; globally, Public Health Care is pathetic!

Even worse news is care of the Humongous Mind. Individual mental healthcare is often accessible only by fortunate individuals and groups even within regions or nations. Mental health care is a significant problem partly because of our misunderstanding about the nature of mental health problems. In particular, we do not distinguish between problems caused by medical diseases and problems induced by the context of life. Worse still, we lack any mechanism whatsoever for dealing with the pathology of the Humongous Mind. There is no genuine world solution for the mass mental illness potentiated by our technologies.

Summary and Message ——————

We have touched on what we have called to Humongous Being and focussed on how our modern technology can facilitate pathology in the Humongous Mind by conveying mis-information and disinformation, the harmful impacts of which are common knowledge. Bad actors have already interfered with elections by publishing false information about candidates and parties. Lies have fomented violence and uprisings. Disinformation has deterred vacci-nation during the recent viral pandemic. False news has prompted the use of drugs with no effect or that are toxic. Malignant misinfor-mation has kindled distrust and hatred and divided people.

Misinformation is clearly a malignant infec-tious disease that we can pass on to one another with horrible consequences, including casual-ties. No wonder that nations use propaganda as a weapon on enemies. Social networks are the primary vector for bringing this 'infectious disease' to the Humongous Mind.

If we choose to listen, we will hear that the Humongous Being has begun to whimper and cry out in its mental distress. There is an intensifying crisis that we can only moderate by deeply understanding the problems our technologies have begotten and fostered, every day affecting more and more of us. It is past the time to act; it is now the time for rescue!

VOLUME 2

Section 4

IN CLOSING

Chapter 20: ——— Final Comments

Addressing mental health in a meaningful and understandable way occupied us for many months over several years. Probably the primary reason for this is that the public social narrative and even the academic literature perseverate in characterizing mental health problems as 'diseases'. This means that they often tell us and expect us to believe that most or all mental problems have a biological origin, and that means they can be treated using classical medical tools like pharmaceuticals and surgery. Worse still is that many people with mental health problems find themselves medicated, perhaps unhelpfully.

It is true that some mental health problems have biological origins, as we have pointed out. However, the vast number of those of us who face mental problems are biologically normal and only the victims of environmental, social or personal dislocations – their problems are normal responses to bad stuff's happening.

If a mental health problem is biological in origin, then intervenors should show the biological signs of the problem, what we call 'biomarkers'. Though we may not have yet discovered a way to properly diagnose some biological causes, it is simply sophistry and wrong to fantasize one and treat that phantasm. Perhaps we can use pharmaceuticals much as we use analgesics to deal with a headache – to relieve the discomfort or sedate – but they do not address the cause of the problem any more than an analgesic cures the headache's cause. Those pharmaceuticals only 'treat' symptoms, and the 'treatment' often is associated with other, sometimes debilitating symptoms and dependencies.

Because of that reality, we (and others) are promoting a paradigm shift, but one absolutely essential to helping all of us who experience the vicissitudes of life. We hope that the shift we target is clear and the result is useful in your thinking. Remember, though: "when it comes paradigms, shift happens"!

Regarding Public Health, it's a different story. When we began writing these books, the Public Health system and the care it provides were on the back burner… and, unfortunately, the burner was set to 'low'. For many years, thought leaders in the health system have promoted the importance of Public Health while governments and other agencies have depopulated the system of professionals. This led to our writing the Dr. Methuselah story. When the COVID-19 pandemic hit and began killing people, there was a metanoia, and we pulled Public Health out of the closet, reanimated it, aired it out and pressed it into essential service. So, writing about Public Health went from being an 'academic' topic to real-world-relevant. That made it worthwhile to invest substantial time and effort in writing about it.

Perhaps our most important message about Public Health is that we still need it. In fact, given the viral threats (and medication-resistant bacteria, fungi and environmental toxins, and…) that are assaulting us, our staying on the green side of the grass is dependent on it! Add to that the points Population Health professionals have made that we must also consider and address the social, economic, nutritional and all the other determinants of health. This means that Public Health must expand its domain. Growing, broadening, populating and maintaining the Public Health system has become mission critical!

We hope you enjoyed the fruits of our efforts and wish you well!

Chapter 21: —————— Summary of Volume 2

In Part 1 of Volume 2, we defined the true nature of mental health problems, clarifying that they are most often not 'illnesses' – biological diseases of the brain – but rather disturbances in thoughts, feelings and behaviors that beset many of us.

We discussed the nature of psychoactive drugs, those that have an impact on the function of the mind, and the general issues associated with pharmaceuticals in mental health care. In choosing a treatment, one must first diagnose what the cause may be. If the cause of the person's mental disturbance is not biological, then the treatment is typically one of the verbal therapies, which have demonstrated significant success. Even when physicians use psychopharmaceuticals, these verbal therapies are valuable, if not essential, adjuncts in returning the patient to a comfortable and functioning state.

We have made our best efforts to describe the body and the brain related to the function of the mind. We emphasize that everything we think, feel, remember and do is determined in our brain that gives birth to our mind. The mind cannot exist without that brain.

We elucidate some of the major psychotherapies and what we as individuals can do in our and others' lives to improve their mental state. We also try to make clear the nature of the complexity of the mind and how things can go wrong within that complex entity.

In its final chapter on mental health, we included some of the views of a psychiatrist regarding how he deals with people with mental health issues.

Part 2 of Volume 2 focused on the nature of Public Health, the care of the populace as a whole. It noted that Public Health has likely made the greatest contributions to the lives of human beings. It accomplished this through centuries of the efforts of key people who found ways to prevent disease and to improve the environment to make it less likely to sicken or even kill us.

At the end of volume 2, we reflect on the COVID-19 Pandemic to illustrate what Public Health is all about.

Why this material is so important, is the fact that we have allowed the public health to wither. We also define the concept of the Humongous Body – the body of bodies of all people – and the Humongous Mind – the reality that we all, to some degree, think, believe and feel together with many others. Interestingly, this work brought us to the issues of misinformation and disinformation and the dangers they pose for communities, countries and even the world.

Chapter 22: ——— What You Can Look to Learn in Volume 1

Introduction ———

We hope that you have found this book on Mental and Public Health to be interesting and full of ideas that are actionable.

Volume 1 is different: it shines light on the health and sickness of the body, called 'physical medicine' and presents the crucial concepts underlying clinical care. This is a brief summary of the most important concepts we address in Volume 1.

This material is crucial as patients, clinicians and others associated with health care must understand it to be able to meaningfully participate in, work with or deal with the professionals, information and processes of health care. The concepts we told you about embody the essence of clinical practice. Understanding them enables those who absorb them to comprehend and critically assess clinical activities and to contribute to their and others' knowledge about clinical care.

However, we can go a step further by noting that someone armed with these concepts and having access to the full range of health information available on the Internet, will be able to understand and solve many clinical problems and evaluate proposed treatments they or their families may encounter.

Let's review them.

The Purposes of Health Care and Medical Visits ———

People visit doctors for only four reasons. They want to (1) feel better, and/or (2) be able to do more, and\or (3) be able to live longer, and/or (4) to learn about their own health. In the latter case, they may wish to get recommendations on how to maintain and improve their health, or to address some administrative purpose, such as getting a doctor's note for insurance, for absences from work, for having missed school, or for immigration or travel documentation.

At every visit, doctors collect information about a patient's comfort and function and may do laboratory investigations to get an estimate of how sick a person is and what their likely longevity is. Based on this information they may intervene if a patient is sick. Health informaticians (professionals who specialize in the creation, management, analysis and use of medical information) and researchers use information management techniques to learn if people are better or worse off after treatment or which types and groups of patients are most likely to experience benefit or harm, feeding this back into clinical care process.

Knowing the purposes of care enables participation in or assessment of the actions of health care teams. This enables answers to important questions. For example: Do the processes and interventions help patients feel better, do more, or live longer? What are the trade-offs patients are prepared to make, such as preferring to avoid cancer chemotherapy because they might prefer a more comfortable life, even if it means shorter survival? When patients are clear about what they expect in terms of changes in comfort, function or life expectancy, clinical teams can design interventions that address patients' personal goals.

Measuring Health

Over the years, experts have developed measures of health. These measures, together with information about a patient's comfort, function, laboratory and imaging findings, help evaluate health status and point to appropriate treatment.

Clinicians, during a visit use these measures, which include qualitative and quantitative information, including symptoms (what a person feels), signs (objective measures from observing a patient or doing tests such as knee reflexes or walking speed) and findings (results from laboratory tests and diagnostic imaging), along with information about an individual's surroundings, to estimate a person's current and future health and the likelihood an intervention will succeed.

There are many health rating scales. 'Measuring Health' by Ian McDowell provides a timeless guide to rating scales and questionnaires that includes some of the many formal systems clinicians use to measure comfort, function and longevity. Knowing how to measure health enables experts on health care teams to evaluate the outcomes of care for individual patients. It also supports clinicians and researchers in developing and using information systems to evaluate clinical care.

We measure the outcomes of care by considering the qualitative and quantitative descriptions of patients before, during and after interventions and using that information to link clinical care to results.

Making a Diagnosis

A diagnosis is an explanation or interpretation of the cause of a problem. Most problems have many possible diagnoses or interpretations. For example, there are at least 3,000 possible diagnoses associated with fatigue. The challenge for clinicians is to develop strategies that enable them to recognize not only common causes for a condition but also rare ones. About 10% of patients have a rare affliction – often ones that are not top of mind for clinicians.

Clinicians must use many techniques to make sure that they have considered all possible causes of a problem before giving up the search. Easily accessible information sources indicate the possible causes of any problem, the additional information necessary to confirm or disprove a diagnosis, and the most effective strategies, questions, examinations and laboratory findings, to pinpoint the correct diagnosis.

DXplain is a medical information system that can help a physician determine the cause (a diagnosis) of a patient's symptoms and findings. Professors use it to teach students about diseases and the strategies they can use to make a diagnosis. DXplain, developed by Dr. Octo Barnett at Massachusetts General Hospital (now part of Mass General Brigham), is only available to credentialed professionals. The reader can try a simpler one, Symptomate (https://symptomate.com/. Accessed Feb.10, 2023) online.

Anyone, including patients, who know what diagnosis is about, can cooperate with a health care team to produce more complete lists of possible causes of patient problems and help to identify the information necessary to confirm or refute a diagnosis. This is especially important when reaching a diagnostic conclusion proves challenging. Patients who work with their healthcare team will feel more confident about abiding medical advice and will recognize when advice might not be appropriate for what they desire or will work in their circumstances.

Evaluating the Usefulness of Tests – False Reassurance, False Alarms, Early Detection and Screening

Physical examination and findings from laboratory tests and medical images produce signals indicating a person's health. Usually, these signals are easy to interpret and suggest a particular health condition or diagnosis. However, occasionally, test results provide false reassurance or incorrectly suggest the presence of a condition that the patient does not have.

False alarms in health care are similar to false alarms for detecting fire: there may be smoke and no fire. False alarms cause needless anxiety and might also produce harm. Just as a fire truck responding to a false fire alarm can be involved in an accident, so a patient can suffer harm when a doctor follows up on a false medical test result alarm. For example, a doctor performing colonoscopy to examine the bowel to follow up on a positive result of stool test (showing blood, a sign of possible colon cancer), might perforate the bowel. Not a good thing if the patient has no disease!

Similarly, men who have a false positive PSA test result for prostate cancer may receive unnecessary and invasive further investigation and intervention, leading to their becoming impotent or incontinent, when the prostate cancer itself would not have harmed them. This is because some prostate cancers grow slowly and will not alter the patient's life expectancy, comfort or function.

The chances of false reassurance or false alarms relate to the characteristics of the tests (sensitivity and specificity, discussed in detail in Section 7) and to the prevalence (frequency of occurrence) of the condition in the population tested. A smoke alarm is more likely to correctly signal for fire in an area with combustible materials. The same is true of a positive test result in people living in an area with a high prevalence of a disease. This means that evaluating the predictive value (accuracy) of a test, we must know not only the characteristics of the test, but also the frequency of the condition in the tested population. For example, a positive test result for an uncommon disease is more likely to be a false alarm than a positive test for a common disease. The predictive value of a test is based on the prevalence (frequency of the condition in the community tested) of the condition, in addition to the

test's sensitivity and specificity, as well as other factors, including the methodology used by the testing laboratory.

Based on all this, it is easy to understand why physicians must repeat certain investigations suggesting the presence of an illness to make sure the test result was meaningful, and why they must follow some tests with other tests that are more specific to an illness. It also makes clear the issues associated with disease screening, which sometimes tests for diseases unlikely for the person's age or situation.

Informaticians track the outcomes of people who have had positive or negative test results in order to produce information about the specificity and sensitivity of tests done by each laboratory.

Biomarkers

Biomarkers are objective (distinct and measurable) findings that provide information about health, illnesses and future health status. Publications have extensive lists of biomarkers and their meanings.

Drugs, both prescription and non-prescription, may also be markers or risk factors predicting the future health of a person. For example, cholesterol lowering drugs may be associated with increased risk of diabetes, and certain antidepressant medications may increase the risk of weight gain, fatigue, or reduced libido.

Issues in Treatment

NNT + NNH

Whenever patients accept treatment recommendations they are making a wager that an intervention is more likely to be helpful than harmful. Almost every treatment helps many people but also harms some.

The standard way of portraying the risk of an intervention, one hardly ever revealed to patients, is a description of The **Numbers**

Needed to Treat and of **The Numbers Needed to Harm**. In other words, how many people must receive a treatment for, on average, one person to benefit (NNT), and how many people who receive a treatment for, on average, one person to experience harm (NNH)?

Relative Risk Reduction

Doctors and patients must also understand the difference between relative risk reduction and absolute risk reduction. Everyone has encountered advertisements claiming that a drug produces a 35% reduction in the risk of harm. Yet, few people understand what this means, and fewer yet understand how the 35% reduction in risk applies to their own circumstance.

One way to understand the difference between absolute and relative risk reduction, is to consider pedestrians crossing a street. People can cross at an intersection or they can jaywalk. The chance of a car hitting a pedestrian is normally very low regardless of whether the person uses a crosswalk or jaywalks. However, in some cities, a person might be twice is likely to be hit when jaywalking. So, the relative risk reduction by using the crosswalk is 50%; a person is 50% less likely to be hit by a car there. However, this might mean that for every 100,000,000 crossings in crosswalks, vehicles will kill one person, while for every 100,000,000 people jaywalking, vehicles will kill two people. Based on these odds, most people would be unlikely to change their behavior. The lifetime risk of a pedestrian-car accident killing someone is quite low: https://www.tnklaw.com/blog-odds-dying-pedestrian-collision/ (Accessed Feb. 10, 2023).

Interventions and Consequences

Doctors may prescribe drugs, but at least a few people experience unintended, moderate to serious consequences. Therefore, measures of the effectiveness of treatments must include an estimate of how the treatment influences sickness or death from any cause, not just the condition the doctor is trying to treat. Consider a treatment to ablate a headache but induces drowsiness. This might or might not be worthwhile for a patient. Knee surgery that successfully cures a knee problem but is associated with a stroke or brain problems from the operation or anesthetic is not necessarily worthwhile.

Accordingly, in evaluating interventions it is important to measure the impact of the treatment on overall health, as well as on the targeted condition, and to have a reasonable estimate of how many people are likely to experience benefit or harm.

The Art of Medicine

Some treatment recommendations are based on objective evidence (e.g., studies and statistics) showing how likely the intervention will benefit or harm a patient. Other treatment recommendations are based on the doctor's knowledge of Biology, Pharmacology and Physiology and represent a 'guesstimate' about which treatment will help. This represents the art of Medicine. Unfortunately, some equally knowledgeable, conscientious and caring clinicians might reach differing conclusions about which intervention is the best, leaving patients and care team members wondering how to resolve the differences in opinion. Reality is that not everything is known or 'computable'. The key is to keep track of what worked and didn't over large numbers of patients.

Another aspect of the art of Medicine is based on the recognition that patients are humans and have needs and feelings. The physician delivers on that by demonstrating listening, caring, empathy and other signs that support patients in their dealing with problems and facing realities.

Other Major Topics ─────────

It is challenging to touch on all of the major content of Volume 1 – only through reading it can one get all of the messages. Here, though, we mention a few of the other topics to give readers some idea of what awaits them when they decide to read Volume 1.

A major issue today, in addition to dealing with biologically based disease, is addressing what is really a sociological disease: Misinformation Disease. Ideas from misinformed or misogynist individuals, who seek either profit or the opportunity to manipulate others, pollute our world. Our approach has been to provide a reasonably good description of what misinformation and disinformation are and how we can protect ourselves from them. We emphasize that the important tactics are to become knowledgeable, seek reliable sources and remain skeptical.

In addition to proffering information about health and health care, we have provided advice on how to go about learning about health. This can be challenging because those who provide care have their own vocabulary and may find it difficult to communicate using terms understandable by patients. Our overall advice regarding the information in these books is to focus on key ideas while leaving the details to when knowing them becomes important to the reader. Towards this objective, we have distinguished between 'Just in Case' learning, typical of how schools approach teaching – by jamming detailed knowledge into learners' heads just in case they may need it. We have suggested, instead, 'Just in Time' learning, where teachers address crucial ideas as their initial focus and instruct students about how to find and learn the details when that becomes important to them.

Throughout the text we have emphasized the importance of evidence: evidence of the various levels of the quality of the information we get. In Medicine, sometimes all that is available is the result of treating a small group of patients with a specific problem. Other times,

researchers have done more formal studies that involved carefully selecting groups of patients and carefully intervening in controlled ways. Interventions not based on evidence of their effectiveness are just shots in the dark and one must rely on luck in terms of outcomes. We point out that the ultimate evidence is in 'systematic reviews' (or meta-analyses). In this latter case, researchers examine and analyze the results of many well structured and carefully executed (randomized and controlled) clinical trials with significant numbers of patients, to tell us what overall will work.

Throughout the text we mention Health Informatics, the discipline that focuses itself on improving health care and the health system, particularly through the use of information, formal processes and computer systems. One of the emphases in Volume 1 is on what Health Informatics has contributed to the development of usable medical records. Regarding those records, we emphasize that their purpose is not just to provide a repository for patient information, but also to serve as the informational basis for analysis and evaluation to ensure that what we do in the health system is worth its substantial cost.

The final matter we will mention related to Volume 1 is that it provides an understanding of the nature of the human beings involved in patient care, including their biases and the possibility of errors. We cite several studies of errors in health care that have shown that patients are injured through misadventures that sometimes were preventable. We show how relatively simple processes can potentially reduce errors and the impacts of human bias, thereby minimizing injuries and saving lives.

Through all of this we emphasize that the intention of clinical care is to help patients, not harm them. Carefulness, mindfulness, critical thinking and acting based on the best evidence available are crucial ways for both physicians and patients to assure that.

Now It is on You! —————————

We leave you with all of this and plus the challenge to use it in your own care and that of your family and friends. For those of you who are in or entering a career that relates to health care, we are confident that this material has prepared you well to really understand clinical care and to use your knowledge as you endeavor to serve!

Chapter 23: ——— What You Can Look Forward to in Volume 3

Personalizing Health Care ———

Among the most interesting and thought stimulating of the three volumes is Volume 3, which addresses crucial knowledge, healthcare problems and solutions and outstanding issues.

This Volume lays out the nature of what occurs, or should occur, when a patient and the doctor meet for the patient's care. It makes it clear that, for this encounter to be successful, trust must exist between the parties, as well as a high degree of intimacy and acceptance, if the patient is to realize the full value of the engagement.

We review the differing levels of seriousness of medical problems and suggest how to go about dealing with them, including some advice about how and when to get advice.

We discuss many medical issues in the volume. These include how to avoid overprescribing, the ethics and principles that must be in place to protect the patient and how to get good information and make rational decisions.

There is a very interesting chapter on death and dying and, though it may sound weird, on how to get sick – primarily so we can all avoid that. We also provide information how the body deals with medications.

Finally, we describe the nature of anesthesia, and include a collection of brief topics that we believe readers will find quite interesting and informative.

Volume 3 is where we collected our thoughts about issues in Medicine. We include what it means to be an expert, and how to confront understanding Medicine – which usually seems to be very challenging area with its own secret language, its own culture and its own cult of high priests, but we can crack its code!

The overall objective of volume 3 is to help all of us think more deeply about Medicine, health care and the people who attempt to help us.

Chapter 24: ———— Writing these Books

Reflections by David (See FIGURE 2.24.1)

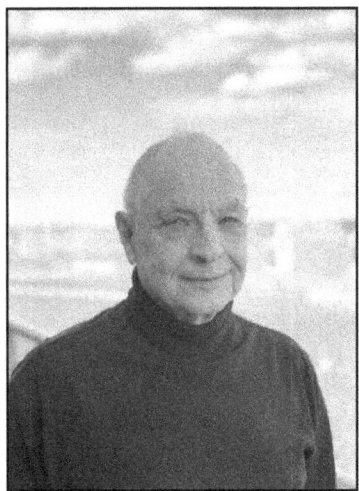

FIGURE 2.24.1: David Zitner

The headlines read "IBM Watson Supercomputer Beats Two Humans at Jeopardy (Feb 2011)".

Computers can record, store and retrieve the world's information. Why wouldn't we expect a thoughtful person using a computer with the world's knowledge at hand to be more effective than people trying to solve problems using only the knowledge in their head? Every thoughtful and empathetic person with access to the world's knowledge can participate in health care – their own and the community's – and contribute to improved health outcomes.

Knowing the essential ideas in clinical care and health services enables each of us to diagnose most problems, evaluate the benefits and harms of proposed remedies, and evaluate and suggest improvements to the proposals of politicians who regulate health care.

Over years of family medical practice, I was startled that even the most sophisticated patients, some with international academic credentials, rarely asked pertinent questions about the care I recommended. They usually accepted my suggestions and did not enquire, even when my recommendation was based on a shaky foundation. They accepted statements without reflection that they would not have accepted in the course of their academic work. On the other hand, a few patients were totally engaged. Even before the Internet, some non-clinicians read the current medical literature and brought me up to date on the recent literature related to their diseases.

Knowledge about health services is becoming increasingly important as each of us becomes more involved in the health services controversies routinely headlined in print and on TV. We dedicated this book to helping people think about health and health care so they can participate in healthcare decisions and become the Chief Executive Officer of their own health care.

I am a retired family doctor, a retired professor in the Division of Medical Education and the founding Director of Medical Informatics at Dalhousie University Medical School, in Halifax, Nova Scotia, Canada. Along with colleagues in Computer Science, I organized and implemented the first Canadian graduate program in Health Informatics.

Half of the students in our graduate program were doctors, nurses, dentists, pharmacists or health educators. The others come from varied backgrounds including Computer

Science, Law, Management, and Engineering and had minimal healthcare experience.

I developed two graduate courses. One, "Health Information Its Flow and Use", tracked the use of information in health care, and addressed how we could use the information normally collected during care to inform health policy and future healthcare decision-making. We dealt with topics, such as what happens to the information collected during clinical encounters and the uses of that information; what happens to the information collected when a doctor examines a patient and recommends treatment; and what happens to the information when a drug either helps someone to heal or when it provokes a serious adverse reaction.

This book is based on another course, "Clinical Care Fundamentals for Non-Clinicians", also known as "learn to think like a doctor and solve medical problems in three months". I developed this course for students who entered the graduate program without any previous healthcare experience. I developed this course so that students could learn how doctors and other health professionals make decisions and which information clinicians need to support their choices.

I was surprised – and so were our students – to find that after 3 months the students were able to solve many medical problems using their brain and a computer, including difficult problems suggested by my doubting clinical colleagues.

Several times a year, students in the course inquired about a diagnosis, test or treatment that doctors prescribed to them, a friend or a family member and they wondered why the doctor suggested it and if it was appropriate.

However, it went beyond that when our inexperienced, "three-month doctors" offered interpretations that were more consistent with modern thinking than the ones the practicing physicians offered. We were especially surprised to find that, in a three-month course, students learned how to choose from various

diagnostic and treatment possibilities and made thoughtful speculations about the causes and treatment of disability and discomfort.

Colleagues at other universities, who heard about our course, including those teaching in other Health Informatics programs, asked for a textbook. Ultimately, this led to these 3 volumes. The material has been adapted to help health services administrators, anyone else pursuing a career in health services, and the general public:

> To understand the purposes of health care

> To consider the many uses of health information

> To consider health policy

> To develop an approach to clinical problems.

Medicine is all about information and knowledge. We all need to ask: Why do I feel sick? Why can't I walk up a flight of stairs? What can I do to prevent and deal with aches, pains, disabilities and the diseases that lead to discomfort, disability and death? Are politicians proposing worthwhile health policies? Are journalistic reports of clinical breakthroughs reasonable or premature?

Those not in health care will benefit from this book because they will learn how doctors make decisions, the questions patients should ask in order to make informed decisions about their own health care, and what we all can do to avoid harm from inappropriate recommendations and medical mistakes.

Graduates of the course understood the purpose of health care; they learned how to diagnose problems, and how to evaluate prospective treatments. You will to!

We expect students, after three months, to use readily available information to understand and solve medical problems. It was a surprise to me that most of our students are able, with the help of a computer, to solve simple and complex medical problems, including dermatology images.

In their final exams our students showed they understood which blood or x-ray tests to use and why, where to find information to tell them all of the possible causes for a particular ache, pain, dysfunction or disability, how to decide what is the most likely cause of a problem, and how to find the right treatment. Our graduates did that, and you, armed with this material, have that potential too.

OUR TARGETS FOR THIS BOOK

1. **The public to help them understand important ideas related to:**
   - *The purposes of health care.*
   - *How the results of care – benefits and harms – are measured.*
   - *Issues around preventive medicine and screening for undiagnosed problems such as breast cancer, cervical cancer (pap smears).*
   - *Deciding if a person has a disease, including how to assess the value of diagnostic tests and procedures. People are surprised to learn that often a positive or negative test result for a disease does not necessarily mean they have or do not have the condition tested for because many tests produce false alarms or false reassurance.*
   - *Assessment of the value of specific treatments, like medications and surgical procedures.*
   - *How interventions can be used to prevent conditions.*
   - *Error prevention and types of errors that can be minimized or avoided.*
   - *Why people with some problems are labeled as being 'mentally ill' while others with similar problems are called 'ill' without the adjective 'mental'.*

2. **Ministries of Health, health services administrators, insurance companies regarding:**
   - *Evaluating health interventions.*
   - *Healthcare resource allocation, including how to measure results and elect among competing demands for resources.*

3. **People working on teams with doctors so that they:**
   - *Have shared and compatible ideas around the purposes of care.*
   - *Can converge on the general and particular approaches to clinical problems.*
   - *Develop ways to resolve differences of opinion among members of healthcare teams.*

Reflections by Dominic (See FIGURE 2.24.2)

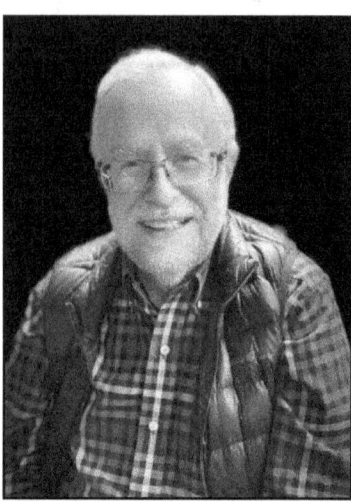

FIGURE 2.24.2: Dominic Covvey

"It's the Journey, not the destination". Stating this often punctuates a disappointing or failed enterprise... sometimes not carried out in one's office! In this case, though, it is a very positive statement about a long writing venture.

David first contacted me about 7 years ago (in Dec 2016) and asked if I wanted to work with him on his interesting and exciting Magnum Opus, his having already put several years into it. He had begun writing a book as a text for his Health Informatics course. I agreed that this might be an interesting way to spend a few months – dramatically misjudging what I faced – as has availed most of my life. We began working and soon mutated and evolved the nature of the end product into something that we hope will have far deeper and broader impacts.

We spent many, many days since that time, writing, editing, repurposing, refining, augmenting and altering the emphasis on many different ideas. The greatest reward in all of this, at least for me, was our communication. We carried out our discussions by telephone across the thousands of kilometers and four hours separating us – we quite literally reach from sea to shining sea! In our discussions, we posited ideas, critiqued them, debated them and both frustrated and delighted each other.

I am not a physician, having started in the areas of Physics, Astrophysics and Medical Biophysics. In the course of my decades of postgraduate study and research in Medicine and immersion in the healthcare system, particularly in cardiovascular research, I picked up a fair amount of medical knowledge. My wife, Carol Thompson, a diagnostic radiologist and ultrasonographer, grandly augmented my experience with Medicine. Regretfully, she exited this mortal coil in 2011, an unendurable loss of the genre the Japanese Emperor said, when he accepted defeat at the end of WW2, we must endure.

Carol taught me a great deal over more than four decades. Some lessons, regretfully, my daughter Beth's dinner guests overheard, turning them disturbingly green! However, being cooked in the soup of Medicine just is not the same as being a clinician who sees patients and diagnoses and treats them,

Since my early research endeavors, I transformed into a health informatician and had the opportunity to work for over 30 years with many different clinicians (including David) and medical groups, as well. Even if you put all that together, clinical medicine is a whole other world. David has been very tolerant of what I claim to know versus what I actually knew. Through discussion, we somehow were able to jointly clarify and even develop novel explanations for some tricky areas, like the nature of health and the mind-brain dichotomy. We also managed to do this despite at times having significant initial disagreements about certain ideas and nuances.

Despite all my limitations, we managed to have what has been one of the most enjoyable intellectual exercises of my career. I have written books previously, back in the 1980s on computer literacy and more recently on esoteric topics like

Health Informatics competencies. The latter contribution was completed in the early 2000s with David and with Bob Bernstein, also a physician (Pointing the Way: Competencies and Curricula in Health Informatics: http://www.nihi.ca/nihi/ir/Pointing%20the%20Way%20MASTER%20Document%20Version%201%20Final.pdf. Relatively speaking, those more recent efforts were intellectually easy and just a lot of hard work. They produced material of interest to only a few thousand people on the planet and, although cited as a contribution, bore none of the satisfaction of the material we share with you.

I have repeatedly heard and learned that the only way to truly understand a topic is to teach it. When we prepare to teach, we often discover that our ideas are ambiguous, incomplete, confused, based on inadequate foundations or just plain wrong. Writing these books has been an exercise like teaching hundreds of classes on the topics of health care and the nature of Medicine. The effort involved in getting the ideas clear enough (albeit never perfectly so – we are mere humans), was enormous and sometimes temporarily insuperable. I hope the effort, with all its near headache-producing intensity, has been worth it for you.

Finally, I wonder if you will be able to extend into your own lives the incredible experience we had. It is my wish that you will read our books and discuss them with your friends, considering, parsing, critiquing and debating the many points we have raised. Book writers probably always hope that people will read what they have written. My hope is that these books will go further and cause you to think about things and explore far beyond what you will find in their pages.

So, I wish you many enjoyable discussions with friends and acquaintances that help you arrive at a place where you see health, health care, and the practice of Medicine for their value and recognize them for their dangers. That will make our effort worth it!

INDEX

Compendium on The Nature of Clinical Care

Volume 1: A Gentle Introduction –

Volume 2: Mental + Public Health Care ————————

Volume 3: Personalizing Health Care ————————